P9-DXE-892

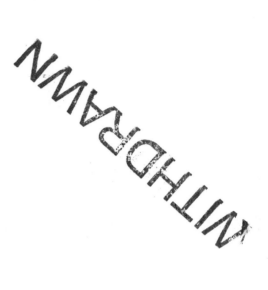

Advance Acclaim for
Me, Myself, and Them

"Like a Sea World underwater view, *Me, Myself, and Them* provides a riveting peek into the world of schizophrenia for parents like me who yearn for understanding. For young people with schizophrenia, like our son, the book orients a frightening illness. For both families and persons with mental illness, this book is laced with hope, something in short supply in most other books."
—*Mindy Greiling, Minnesota State Representative and Executive Board Member, National Alliance on Mental Illness*

"The firsthand account is realistic."
—*Jim Greiling, diagnosed with schizophrenia at age 21, now 29 years old*

"This beautifully told personal story provides an innovative platform for solid information about schizophrenia and its treatment. Highly informative to persons struggling with the onset of psychosis, and to families, friends, and mental health workers who struggle to understand and help."
—*William T. Carpenter Jr., M.D., Professor of Psychiatry and Pharmacology, University of Maryland School of Medicine*

"The authors provide a first rate resource for anyone whose life is touched by schizophrenia. Through solid, easy to understand language, the manuscript provides useful guidance for others coping with this disease. Highly recommended."
—*Ming Tsuang, M.D., Ph.D., Department of Psychiatry, University of California, San Diego*

"*Me, Myself, and Them: A Firsthand Account of One Young Person's Experience with Schizophrenia* is a straightforward and marvelously lucid retelling of Kurt Snyder's battle with his demons. Not only does it show us the experience of psychosis, it also explains, in jargon-free language, what each element of that experience means. Compelling and eminently readable, a book like this ought to be required reading for all high school and college students, demystifying as it does an illness all too long shrouded in misunderstanding, confusion and fear."
—*Pamela Spiro Wagner, author of* Divided Minds: Twin Sisters and Their Journey Through Schizophrenia

"I strongly recommend this book to patients, families, clinicians, and researchers interested in a firsthand account of how schizophrenia changes the way the world looks, feels, and behaves. It is very moving and very informative. From compelling descriptions of changes in mood, cognition, and perception to explanations about how the brain is affected and how drugs work, this brief but detailed personal statement and review of the state of the field is invaluable."
—*Daniel R. Weinberger, M.D., Director, Genes, Cognition and Psychosis Program IRP, NIMH, NIH*

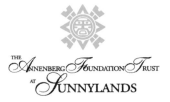

THE
ᏘNNENBERG ℱOUNDATION ᏘRUST
AT ᏘUNNYLANDS

The Annenberg Foundation Trust at Sunnylands'
Adolescent Mental Health Initiative

Patrick E. Jamieson, Ph.D., *series editor*

Me, Myself, and *Them*

A Firsthand Account of One Young Person's Experience With Schizophrenia

Kurt Snyder

with Raquel E. Gur, M.D., Ph.D., and Linda Wasmer Andrews

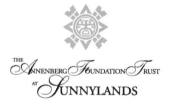

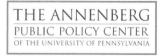

The Annenberg Foundation Trust at Sunnylands'
Adolescent Mental Health Initiative

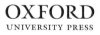

THE ANNENBERG
PUBLIC POLICY CENTER
OF THE UNIVERSITY OF PENNSYLVANIA

OXFORD
UNIVERSITY PRESS

2007

OXFORD
UNIVERSITY PRESS

Oxford University Press, Inc., publishes works that further
Oxford University's objective of excellence
in research, scholarship, and education.

The Annenberg Foundation Trust at Sunnylands
The Annenberg Public Policy Center of the University of Pennsylvania
Oxford University Press

Oxford   New York
Auckland   Cape Town   Dar es Salaam   Hong Kong   Karachi
Kuala Lumpur   Madrid   Melbourne   Mexico City   Nairobi
New Delhi   Shanghai   Taipei   Toronto

With offices in
Argentina   Austria   Brazil   Chile   Czech Republic   France   Greece
Guatemala   Hungary   Italy   Japan   Poland   Portugal   Singapore
South Korea   Switzerland   Thailand   Turkey   Ukraine   Vietnam

Library of Congress Cataloging-in-Publication Data
Snyder, Kurt.
Me, myself, and them : a firsthand account of one young person's experience with
schizophrenia / by Kurt Snyder with Raquel E. Gur, and Linda Wasmer Andrews.
    p. cm.—(Adolescent mental health initiative)
"The Annenberg Foundation Trust at Sunnylands, the Annenberg Public Policy Center."
Includes bibliographical references and index.
ISBN 978-0-19-531123-5; 978-0-19-531122-8 (pbk)
1. Snyder, Kurt—Mental health.   2. Schizophrenics—United States—Biography.
3. Schizophrenia in adolescence—United States.   I. Gur, Raquel E.   II. Andrews, Linda
Wasmer.   III. Title.
RC514.S565A3 2007
616.89'80092–dc22   2007016619

9   8   7   6   5   4   3   2   1

Printed in the United States of America
on acid-free paper

Contents

Three
In the Grip of *Them*: Losing Touch With Reality 53

Four
Naming and Facing the Enemy: Diagnosis and Treatment 79

Foreword

The Adolescent Mental Health Initiative (AMHI) was
created by The Annenberg Foundation Trust at Sunnylands to share with mental health professionals, parents, and
adolescents the advances in treatment and prevention now
available to adolescents with mental health disorders. The Initiative was made possible by the generosity and vision of
Ambassadors Walter and Leonore Annenberg, and the project
was administered through the Annenberg Public Policy Center
of the University of Pennsylvania in partnership with Oxford
University Press.

The Initiative began in 2003 with the convening, in Philadelphia and New York, of seven scholarly commissions made
up of over 150 leading psychiatrists and psychologists from
around the country. Chaired by Drs. Edna B. Foa, Dwight L.
Evans, B. Timothy Walsh, Martin E. P. Seligman, Raquel E.
Gur, Charles P. O'Brien, and Herbert Hendin, these commissions were tasked with assessing the state of scientific research on the prevalent mental disorders whose onset occurs
predominantly between the ages of 10 and 22. Their collective

findings now appear in a book for mental health professionals and policy makers titled *Treating and Preventing Adolescent Mental Health Disorders* (2005). As the first product of the Initiative, that book also identified a research agenda that would best advance our ability to prevent and treat these disorders, among them anxiety disorders, depression and bi-polar disorder, eating disorders, substance abuse, and schizo-phrenia.

The second prong of the Initiative's three-part effort is a series of smaller books for general readers. Some of the books are designed primarily for parents of adolescents with a specific mental health disorder. And some, including this one, are aimed at adolescents themselves who are struggling with a mental illness. All of the books draw their scientific informa-tion in part from the AMHI professional volume, presenting it in a manner that is accessible to general readers of different ages. The "teen books" also feature the real-life story of one young person who has struggled with—and now manages—a given mental illness. They serve as both a source of solid re-search about the illness and as a roadmap to recovery for afflicted young people. Thus they offer a unique combination of medical science and firsthand practical wisdom in an effort to inspire adolescents to take an active role in their own recovery.

The third part of the Sunnylands Adolescent Mental Health Initiative consists of two Web sites. The first, www.Cope CareDeal.org, addresses teens. The second, www.oup.com/ us/teenmentalhealth, provides updates to the medical com-munity on matters discussed in *Treating and Preventing Adolescent Mental Health Disorders*, the AMHI professional book.

We hope that you find this volume, as one of the fruits of the Initiative, to be helpful and enlightening.

Patrick Jamieson, Ph.D.
Series Editor
Adolescent Risk Communication Institute
Annenberg Public Policy Center
University of Pennsylvania
Philadelphia, PA

Preface

Hi. My name is Kurt Snyder. I'm 34 years old and I have schizophrenia. I live just outside Annapolis, Maryland, in the United States.

I developed schizophrenia gradually over a period of about ten years, beginning when I was about 18 years old. For most of that time, none of my family or friends realized I was having mental problems. Eventually, however, my symptoms became severe, and then everyone noticed there was something wrong with me. I started to think I was under surveillance 24 hours a day by some unseen group of people. At one point, I wondered whether my whole life was manufactured by some type of virtual reality machine, operated by aliens.

While I was ill, I couldn't work effectively. I tried working part time, but I was fired from two different jobs within a month. I became very depressed, and for a while, I had no mental energy whatsoever. I couldn't even rake leaves in my own backyard. I started to realize that I was having mental problems, that my brain was broken. I thought I was never going to be able to do any productive work ever again. I thought I would never achieve anything significant, and my friends would drift away from me. I thought I was inadequate for life. I expected to live out the rest of my days in sorrow and misery.

I was wrong.

That was six years ago. Today, I have been working effectively at the same job for the last four years. I'm a database administrator (a computer-related job) employed by the state of Maryland. I am also president of my local volunteer fire department, which I joined six years ago. All my friends have stayed with me. With the help of medication, my illness is in remission. I have had only minimal symptoms of schizophrenia over the last three years.

I'm writing this book to help you understand one thing: Having schizophrenia is not a death sentence. Life goes on, sometimes better than you might have hoped. You may be having a difficult time dealing with the symptoms and expression of this disease, whether it's you or someone you know who has schizophrenia. However, these difficult times may not be permanent. If you are willing to work hard toward a successful outcome, in many cases the symptoms of schizophrenia can be managed and controlled. The life of a person with schizophrenia can grow and develop just as that of anyone else who doesn't have this disease.

How This Book Came to Be

There are a number of books about schizophrenia in print, but few are written especially for teenagers and young adults. Fewer still are first-person accounts of what it really feels like to fight schizophrenia and win. This book aims to fill that void.

The idea for the book started with seven scholarly commissions on adolescent mental health that were convened in 2003 by the Annenberg Foundation Trust at Sunnylands. The psychiatrists and psychologists on these commissions were charged with looking at the state of the science on mental disorders that strike teenagers and young adults. Several books about adolescent mental health followed, including the one you hold in your hands.

The chair of the schizophrenia commission was Raquel E. Gur, M.D., Ph.D., who also is medical adviser and coauthor for this book. Dr. Gur is Professor of Psychiatry, Neurology, and Radiology at the University of Pennsylvania. In addition, she has acted as director of the Neuropsychiatry Section and the Schizophrenia Research Center there. Her career has been devoted to studying brain function in schizophrenia, so she brings a wealth of experience and expertise to these pages.

The third person on our writing team is Linda Wasmer Andrews, a journalist who has specialized in writing about mental health issues for more than two decades. One of the ways that she contributed to the book was by interviewing other people who struggled with schizophrenia in their teens and twenties. You'll see their stories sprinkled throughout these pages in sidebars titled "Other Faces of Schizophrenia." To protect the privacy of interview participants, pseudonyms are used. But their stories, often told in their own words, are true, honest, and filled with helpful hints and hopeful insights. I've also used pseudonyms for the rest of the people who appear in this book. All of the events I describe are 100% true.

What You'll Find Here

Together, my coauthors and I have teamed up to create a unique book that looks at schizophrenia from multiple points of view. It's the firsthand account of my battle to overcome schizophrenia, but it's also the story of the other 2.4 million Americans—and the 24 million people worldwide—who have this feared yet fascinating disease.

To give you a broader perspective on topics such as causes, symptoms, diagnosis, treatment, and self-management, we've divided each chapter into two parts. First comes my personal account of living with schizophrenia. Then comes a jointly written section called "The Big Picture," which looks at the science, medicine, and social trends that affect not only me, but perhaps also you.

One of the more interesting things about schizophrenia is the diversity of forms it can take. I have paranoid schizophrenia, which is characterized by distorted thoughts and perceptions that sometimes center around the belief that others are "out to get you." As a result, this form of the disease will be described in the most detail here. However, we'll also discuss other forms at lesser length. And much of the information about diagnosis, treatment, and coping strategies is applicable to anyone with schizophrenia, regardless of the particular way it manifests itself.

I invite you to read my story and gain some insight into the life of a person who suffered for years with schizophrenia, but has now recovered and is leading a normal life. If you are currently experiencing symptoms, I hope that I might be able to offer some guidance and help direct you toward a brighter future, where mental disease doesn't dictate the type of life you lead.

Me, Myself, and *Them*

Chapter One

A Fragmented Mind: Overview of Schizophrenia

My Story

I first started to experience what I believe were definite symptoms of schizophrenia in college. Some of these symptoms may have been triggered by the new environment, as a reaction to a new lifestyle. My first semester was rather unremarkable—my grades were very good and I seemed to handle classes well. Everything fell apart during my second semester, when I became disorganized, lost my concentration during class, and failed to complete many of my homework assignments. I ended the year with very poor grades. The following semester wasn't much better. I eventually lost an academic scholarship I had earned in high school.

Delusions of Grandeur

Sometime during that first year, I started having a common symptom of mental illness—grandiose thinking. I believed that I was going to discover some fabulous new mathematical principle that would transform the way we view the universe. I told no one about these thoughts. I started looking for clues to this mathematical theory in math books I found at the library.

I actually learned very little about math though, because I couldn't focus on any of the material for any significant length of time. I couldn't digest what I was reading. But I still thought that one day I would get a flash of inspiration and become famous. I spent hours every day daydreaming, trying to think of new undiscovered relationships between numbers, symbols, and the objects of the real world. I told myself I was always on the verge of discovery, and I hadn't discovered the right idea because I just wasn't thinking hard enough. I knew it would take a genius to solve some of the problems I was thinking about, but I didn't realize that I wasn't a genius. I was over-estimating my own abilities. Because of this preoccupation with numbers, I did very poorly in college over the next two years.

During my third year of college, I developed other symptoms more closely related to paranoid schizophrenia. Once, I saw a police car behind me, and I thought the police were following me. This concern lasted for perhaps an hour or more, even after the police car had disappeared in traffic. Later in the year, I went on a short vacation with my brother, his wife, and my girlfriend in the mountains of western Maryland. We rented a house in the woods for a weekend. One evening, I suddenly started to feel very vulnerable and helpless. I imagined that someone might break into the house while we were asleep and kill us all. I don't know that I communicated much of what I was thinking to my companions, but I was very concerned about the sturdiness of the entrance doors, and they noticed that I was strangely preoccupied. Eventually, I calmed down and went to bed. Later on in that year, the symptoms of paranoia returned when

I cut my leg and decided to go to the university medical clinic. While I was there, I started to feel very vulnerable. I wondered if the nurses would try to hurt me in some way and I tried to imagine how they might do this. I thought they might try to infect me with the AIDS virus by using a tainted needle.

These symptoms were not only irrational, but also indicated extreme paranoia. Thankfully, the episodes were brief, and did not significantly affect my thought processes for more than a few hours. Several more years would pass before I exhibited paranoid symptoms again.

Even though my paranoia was short lived at this time, disorganization continued to be a problem for me. I found that my thoughts and my behaviors were erratic. For example, I would plan to go to class, then on my way there I would decide to go somewhere else—the gym perhaps. While on my way to the gym, I would decide to get something to eat instead. But before reaching the dining hall, I might decide to stop at the library. I would change my mind again and again, often several times within a few minutes. My whole day would be spent going here and there, but getting nowhere, and certainly not accomplishing anything productive.

One side of this thought disorganization was forgetfulness. I would misplace important objects, like my keys or wallet. I couldn't remember where I put them. I laid them down some-place haphazardly without thinking about what I was doing, searching frantically later when I needed them again. I lost books, articles of clothing, pens—anything—even my car. I would park my car somewhere on campus and then forget where it was, sometimes not even remembering which parking lot it was in. Luckily for me, my car at that time was an old, bright reddish-orange Toyota Corolla. It was easy to see, so it didn't usually take me a long time to find it.

Eventually, continued lack of academic success in college convinced me that I was not a good student. I decided to go to school part time, and I changed my major from engineering to hotel management, something I considered much less challenging. The new major was much easier for me. The classes I had to take for hotel management required much less concentration, and much less homework. My grades improved significantly. I continued going to school part-time for two or three years, taking one or two classes per semester. In the end however, I decided that I wanted to work for myself on a permanent basis, and that I didn't want the type of career that a college education promised. I decided to create a job for myself. I would strike out as an entrepreneur. I'll tell you more about that later in the book.

The Early Days

I can't think of anything in my childhood or teenage years that could have predicted mental illness in me. I did not have any childhood experiences that would normally be considered traumatic. My childhood, for the most part, was very nice. I grew up in a residential neighborhood just south of Baltimore City, in Maryland. I had one brother who was almost four years older than I. We played together often, but of course he was always stronger, faster, and better than I at any physical activity. I often longed for the day when I could beat him at soccer, basketball, wrestling, running, swimming, whatever. I also had a best friend, Chris, who was my constant companion. We saw each other nearly every day. We became "blood brothers" one summer, pricking our fingers and shaking hands on the blood to seal the deal.

Growing up, sports and school were the most important elements in my life. I tried to play baseball one season, but I was not a natural talent and I quickly tired of it. Soccer was the real highpoint of my athletic activities. I was much better at it than baseball or basketball. My father coached my soccer team one year, and Chris was part of the team. I remember that was a real treat.

My mother and father were always very encouraging in everything I did, whether it was school, sports, or anything else. They supported my brother and me in all possible ways. For the most part, I felt loved, secure, and safe at home. Our extended family was also very supportive. My grandmother on my mother's side and her sister, my great aunt, visited us nearly every week. They took care of me and my brother when we were sick, and took us on special trips on the weekends and in the summertime. My grandparents on my father's side lived about two hours away in Pennsylvania. We saw them often also. I grew up with the sense that family values and family relationships were important, and I learned good moral values as a child that have stayed with me my whole life. I knew that my parents and my family loved me.

In elementary school, I did very well, from an academic standpoint. I always scored high on standardized tests. I was well behaved and well liked by my teachers. Upon graduation from the sixth grade, I earned a good citizenship award, given to a single student out of a graduating class of about 75 students total. I was very proud of this award.

Even though I had a best friend, played sports, and did well in school, I didn't have many other friends my age. In elementary school, I didn't seem to form personal bonds with other students in my class. I was shy and reserved among my peers, and I also had a poor self-image.

...I didn't seem to form personal bonds with other students in my class.

I didn't feel worthwhile. This self-concept certainly wasn't a result of mom or dad's parenting behavior.

Part of my poor self-image resulted from two experiences I had during elementary school, which caused me great shame for several years. These two experiences were prominent in my thoughts for a long time. I don't know why they affected me for so long, but it is clear to me that I wasn't emotionally mature enough to healthfully deal with these experiences.

The first occurred while I was in second grade. My parents had entered me in a track meet for children. The race was about to begin and I was standing on the track with several other kids when suddenly I felt the need to go to the bathroom. I couldn't hold back the tide and I wet my pants while waiting for the race to start, in plain sight of everyone there. My mom promptly took me out of the race. "Why didn't you say something to us? Why didn't you say you had to go to the bathroom?" she said. I honestly don't know why. But the embarrassment I felt lasted all day, all month, all year, and for several years afterward. I think the emotional reaction I had to this experience and the continued effect it had on me was abnormal. Most kids probably would have gotten over it rather quickly.

The other incident occurred in the fourth or fifth grade. At that time, Chris's mother was picking us up from school every day. One day, instead of waiting for us in the school parking lot, she decided to go into school to talk to one of the teachers. She left her van unlocked so we could go out and wait for her.

Earlier that day, I had had a dispute with some other kids in my class. Two or three of them followed me out to the van and stole my book bag, refusing to give it back to me. I became afraid and decided to get in the van instead of facing these children. This was uncharacteristic of me, because normally I was not a fearful child, and I didn't usually back down from a confrontation with other kids. Although Chris was there with me, he was small for his age, and I didn't think he would be much help. I suppose I felt vulnerable because I was outnumbered. Eventually, Chris's mother came out to the van, I got my bag back, and we went home. However, I felt ashamed that I did not stand up to these children. This shame weighed heavily on me for several years. It developed into feelings of inadequacy and inferiority. I became more introverted and reluctant to interact with my peers, and I avoided contact with other kids in my class. These feelings of inadequacy influenced me well into adulthood, and affected my ability to form friendships with other teenagers—especially girls.

I never talked to my parents, my friends, or anyone else about feeling inferior. I kept these thoughts to myself. I wanted to bury them in a hole and be rid of them forever. Of course, they only continued to fester inside me. I realize now that keeping things to yourself is a mistake. It is almost always better to discuss your concerns with other people. If I had done that in elementary school, perhaps I wouldn't have lived for years with such a negative view of myself.

In high school, I was mostly quiet and withdrawn. I still enjoyed sports, playing soccer and lacrosse, and wrestling. I was probably best in wrestling, and became physically fit due to wrestling practice.

I dated little. I was afraid to express myself to girls, probably because of my negative self-perception, and an associated lack of confidence. I was self-conscious. The girls in my school knew me as a quiet person, and so naturally, most of them did not approach me. I wasn't popular.

In the eleventh grade I received a big boost of confidence when I went on a student exchange trip. A select group of students from my school went to Italy for three weeks, and each of us lived with an Italian family and went to an Italian school. Soon, I found that the Italian girls were interested in me! Not just one, but several! They didn't know me as the shy, reserved boy I was in the United States. I attracted one very good-looking Italian girl who spent the day with me in Venice. It was my good luck that not far from Piazza San Marco I kissed a girl for the first time in my life. It was wonderful! When I came back to the States, I was a changed boy, if only a little bit.

I ended my high school career with good grades, several academic awards, a college scholarship, and optimism for the future.

The Big Picture

Schizophrenia. The word itself sounds harsh and forbidding. We've all heard the word, of course, and most of us have a vague idea of what it means. But you never think it will happen to you—until one day it does.

The truth is, schizophrenia can strike anyone. It's a disease like any other, based in biological processes gone awry. And like many other serious, long-term diseases, this one has wide-ranging consequences—mentally, emotionally, physically, and socially. Yet there's something about schizophrenia that sets it apart. Compared to heart disease or diabetes, for example, schizophrenia seems to inspire more confusion, misinformation, and exaggerated fear. This book certainly isn't going to downplay the challenges of the disease. They are very real and often quite formidable, as you'll read in these pages. However, you'll also read about how the challenges can often be met with time, effort, and the right treatment and support services.

So What Is Schizophrenia?

The word *schizophrenia* literally means "fragmented mind." Contrary to what you may have heard, that's not the same thing as a "split personality." When you have schizophrenia, you don't have multiple personalities warring inside your head. Instead, you have a single personality, but a mind that has shattered. Thoughts, feelings, and behaviors break apart into disconnected bits.

The Real "Split Personality"

Dissociative identity disorder (also called multiple personality disorder) is a form of mental illness in which people have two or more distinct identities. These identities take turns controlling the person's behavior. Each identity may have its own name, personality traits, and self-image. Some identities may not remember what the others did, which can lead to large, unexplained gaps in the person's memory. Dissociative identity disorder is *not* a form of schizophrenia, but rather a separate disorder with an entirely different set of causes, symptoms, and treatments.

Schizophrenia is a severe and long-lasting mental disorder. It can impair the ability to think clearly, which in turn can impair the ability to speak coherently and behave in a way that makes sense to other people. For instance, some people with the disorder believe that others are reading their minds or controlling their thoughts, and their words and actions reflect these distorted beliefs.

Schizophrenia also can make it hard to distinguish what's real from what isn't. People with the disease sometimes hear voices or see things that aren't really there. For some, schizophrenia also reduces the ability to express emotions and feel enjoyment. For others, it drains away all energy and motivation.

Not surprisingly, such drastic changes in how the mind works can touch every corner of a person's existence. People with schizophrenia may have trouble making decisions, managing their emotions, and relating to others. If the disease is left untreated, they may have great difficulty going to school, holding down a job, or living on their own as adults. Yet the picture isn't as bleak as it might sound. While the symptoms may never totally disappear, they often can be managed by getting proper treatment and learning strategies for living with the disease. Once, schizophrenia was a dire diagnosis that held little hope for recovery. Today, many people with schizophrenia do indeed get better and go on to lead full, productive, satisfying lives.

Ancient Illness or Modern Scourge?

Schizophrenia is not a new problem, but there is still some debate about when the disease made its first appearance in recorded history. Mental illness in general has been recognized for many thousands of years. In ancient Greece, it was sometimes ascribed to an imbalance of bodily fluids, and in medieval Europe, it was often blamed on demonic possession.

The specific symptoms that characterize schizophrenia were not widely described until the early 1800s, however. Scholars differ in their explanation for this lapse. Some believe that schizophrenia was always there, but was not differentiated from other forms of mental illness or was seen as divine intervention rather than a disease. Others believe that schizophrenia truly was rare until the 1800s, when it suddenly appeared in its modern form.

Who Gets Schizophrenia?

Most people who develop schizophrenia have their first episode as older teenagers or young adults. The disease is very rare before age 13, affecting only about 1 in 40,000 children. It's more common but still unusual in teens younger than 18. In adults ages 18 and older, however, schizophrenia strikes about 1 in 100 people.

Schizophrenia tends to start earlier in males than in females. The peak time for schizophrenia to appear is the late teens through early twenties for men, compared to the mid-twenties through early thirties for women. It seldom starts after age 45. Overall, the disease affects men and women about equally.

Schizophrenia is found in ethnic groups around the globe. In fact, the World Health Organization estimates that the disease affects about 24 million people worldwide. While great strides in treatment have been made in developed countries such as the United States, the majority of people with schizophrenia in developing countries still aren't receiving the medical care they need.

Where Does Schizophrenia Come From?

Scientists are still studying the exact causes of schizophrenia. Like many other illnesses, though, this one is thought to be caused by a combination of genetic, environmental, and biological forces. These three forces interact in complicated ways. Genes alone probably aren't enough to cause schizophrenia. However, they may make a person more vulnerable to certain stresses and strains in the environment that can set the disease

...the ultimate source of many symptoms seems to lie in a person's brain chemistry, structure, and function.

in motion. Whatever the trigger, the ultimate source of many symptoms seems to lie in a person's brain chemistry, structure, and function.

THE ROLE OF GENETICS

Scientists have long known that schizophrenia runs in families. About 1% of the general adult population has the disorder. But about 10% of individuals with a parent, brother, or sister who has schizophrenia will go on to develop the disorder, too. The risk is highest for those with an identical twin who has schizophrenia. Such individuals have a 40% to 65% chance of developing the disease as well.

Progress has been made in identifying genes that are associated with schizophrenia. However, each gene seems to have a small impact, and none seems able to cause the disease all by itself. Scientists are still unable to predict which individuals will get schizophrenia from their genetic makeup alone.

THE ROLE OF THE ENVIRONMENT

Even among people whose identical twins have schizophrenia, 35% to 60% remain free of the disease. Clearly, something other than just genetics is affecting their risk. To determine what that "something else" might be, scientists have looked at factors in the environment. Among the possible risk factors that have been identified are exposure to viruses or injury during pregnancy as well as problems during birth, any of which might lead to changes in the developing brain.

Another possible contributing factor is exposure to stressful life experiences. However, researchers studying this link often run into difficulty when they try to sort cause from effect. Let's say a person with schizophrenia is living in poverty. Do stressful living conditions contribute to that individual's symptoms? Perhaps. But the symptoms also may make it hard for the person to keep a job, which certainly contributes to being impoverished. In cases such as this, there often is no clear-cut answer to the question of which came first, the disease or the life stress.

Fifty years ago, many mental health professionals believed that the roots of schizophrenia could be traced back to bad parenting. Mothers got a particularly bad rap. In more recent decades, however, theories pointing the finger at parents have been largely debunked. None have held up to the scrutiny of scientific research. While some families are undeniably more stressful to live in than others, there's no evidence that bad parenting per se means you will develop schizophrenia—just as there's no evidence that good parenting guarantees you won't. In truth, many people with schizophrenia come from close, loving homes. And even when family relationships are more troubled, it's difficult to untangle the causes of the disease from the problems caused by it.

IMBALANCES IN BRAIN CHEMISTRY

The human brain contains about one hundred billion neurons, nerve cells that are specially designed to send information to other nerve, muscle, or gland cells. Every neuron is separated from each of its neighbors by a tiny gap called a synapse. This gap serves as the site where information is relayed from one neuron to the next. On average, each neuron makes synaptic connections with one thousand other neurons. In total, then, it's estimated that there are between one hundred trillion and one quadrillion synapses in the brain—numbers so large they're almost impossible to contemplate.

To send a message to its neighbors, a neuron must rely on chemical messengers called neurotransmitters to ferry the message across the synaptic space. It works like this: The sending neuron releases a neurotransmitter into the synapse. There are more than one hundred different kinds of neurotransmitters in the brain, and each has its own distinctive shape. A particular type of neurotransmitter can only dock with its receptor, a matching molecule on the surface of the receiving neuron. Once this happens, the neurotransmitter can deliver its message.

Schizophrenia seems to be related to imbalances in various neurotransmitters. Among those that may play a key role in the disorder are dopamine, serotonin, gamma-amino-butyric acid (GABA), and glutamate.

- Dopamine is a neurotransmitter that is essential for movement and also influences motivation and perception of reality. Some antipsychotic medications seem to work by blocking dopamine receptors. According to one hypothesis, symptoms such as confused thinking and auditory hallucinations might be caused by excessive dopamine activity in the brain. Another hypothesis states that symptoms such as lack of motivation and interest might be caused by the breakdown of dopamine into other chemicals over time. Whatever the case, dopamine doesn't seem to be the sole cause of schizophrenia, since not everyone with the disorder has an increased number of dopamine receptors. It's also possible that some changes in the brain's dopamine circuits might be an effect of schizophrenia rather than a cause.
- Serotonin is a neurotransmitter that helps regulate mood, sleep, appetite, and sexual drive. Some researchers suspect that schizophrenia may be related to an excess of serotonin in the brain. This is the reverse of depression and anxiety, both of which have been linked to low levels of serotonin.
- GABA is a neurotransmitter that inhibits the flow of nerve signals in neurons by blocking the release of other neurotransmitters. Glutamate is another neurotrans-

mitter with the opposite function; it promotes the flow of nerve signals in neurons. Researchers now believe that schizophrenia may involve significant abnormalities in these two chemicals, as well. One possibility is that glutamate may be overly active in part of the brain responsible for complex thought, and symptoms such as an apparent lack of motivation and interest are really just a defense against overstimulation.

ABNORMALITIES IN BRAIN STRUCTURE AND FUNCTION

Scientists have used sophisticated imaging techniques to compare the brains of people with schizophrenia to those of healthy individuals. Several differences have been noted, although the significance of these differences is still not entirely clear. For example, some people with schizophrenia have enlarged ventricles, fluid-filled cavities inside the brain. Others have a smaller-than-average hippocampus, part of the brain involved in emotion, learning, and memory.

The prefrontal cortex is part of the brain involved in complex thought, problem solving, and judgment. These mental functions are typically affected by schizophrenia, so you might expect that the prefrontal cortex would be affected, too. Indeed, studies have found that schizophrenia may be associated with unusual activity, decreased size, or abnormal development in this area. Yet while such differences are found in many people with schizophrenia, they're subtle and not present in everyone.

Although there is still much to learn, one thing seems clear: It's unlikely that researchers will ever pinpoint a single cause for such a complex disease. Instead, schizophrenia seems to

It's also possible that what we now call schizophrenia could turn out to be not one disease but several...

result from the interaction of multiple factors. It's also possible that what we now call schizophrenia could turn out to be not one disease but several, each with its own combination of genetic, environmental, and biological causes.

What Are the Early Warning Signs?

The first hints of trouble are often subtle. The term *prodromal* refers to preliminary symptoms of schizophrenia that may appear two to six years before the first major episode occurs. Such symptoms may include:

- Reduced ability to concentrate and pay attention
- Decreased energy and motivation
- Mood changes, such as depression and anxiety
- Irritability
- Sleep problems
- Social withdrawal
- Suspiciousness
- Neglect of personal appearance
- Drop in school performance
- Loss of interest in activities previously enjoyed

The difficulty with these symptoms is that they're so vague. Almost everyone has mild problems with some of these symptoms, some of the time. Even when the symptoms are more severe and troublesome, they frequently are signs of a more common disorder, such as depression or substance abuse. Most teenagers who have these symptoms never go on to develop schizophrenia. And to make matters more confusing, young people who *do* later develop schizophrenia don't necessarily have all these symptoms in the years leading up to their first major episode.

Other Faces of Schizophrenia: "Mark"

Today Mark is a 29-year-old mental health advocate who lives alone, works part time, and has a serious girlfriend. Getting to this point didn't come without a struggle, however. When Mark was 16, he began suffering from depression. "I thought it was due to other things that were going on in my life," he recalls. "In junior high school, I was a poor student. I had a reputation for being smart, but I didn't apply myself, and I didn't get along with my teachers. Then right before I hit high school, I made a pact with myself that I was going to buckle down and get serious."

At first, everything seemed to be going according to plan. Mark was doing well despite taking challenging subjects such as Latin, and he had set some lofty goals for himself: to become president of the honor society and get accepted by Harvard. "By the time I was 16, though, I could see that I was not going to reach my goals," he says. "I became heavily depressed. At the time, I thought it was just depression brought on by my failure, but now I think there was something biological going on."

Mark didn't get into Harvard, but he did receive a scholarship to another university. Unfortunately, the long slide just continued in college. He found it impossible to focus on his studies, so his grades fell and his scholarship eventually was revoked. Then at age 18, Mark had a major episode that ended with him "shouting, screaming, and naked" in the college chapel. "I thought the CIA was trying to recruit me," he recalls. "I was really scared and confused, so I went to the chapel, because it was a place where I'd found a lot of strength in the past. It sounds crazy, but I was afraid I was going to get shot. I remembered reading somewhere that if you're naked they won't shoot you. So I took off my clothes so they wouldn't think I had a weapon."

At the hospital afterward, Mark was diagnosed with schizoaffective disorder, a condition that combines the distorted thoughts and perceptions of schizophrenia with severe disturbances in mood. In hindsight, it's easy to find the seeds of this disorder in Mark's earlier depression. At the time, though, it wasn't so clear. Depressed feelings are very common, and for the large majority of teenagers, they don't herald either schizophrenia or schizoaffective disorder. Mark had no way of knowing that he would wind up in the minority until that day in the university chapel.

"Even afterward, I didn't want to believe it—denial is a big deal," says Mark. "I had to come to grips with the fact that there was something mentally wrong with me. It wasn't just that people didn't understand me or I was having a bad few days." Eventually, however, Mark came to terms with his diagnosis. And in the years since, he has slowly but surely glued the pieces of his life back together.

It's often only in retrospect that the true significance of these early symptoms becomes apparent. Over time, though, the warning signs evolve into something more distressing and disruptive. A person might start hearing voices that aren't there, believing that newscasters on TV are talking directly to him, or thinking that he can do harm to others just by looking at them. Eventually, these kinds of disordered thoughts and perceptions are bound to result in behavior that seems extremely odd to other people. By this point, it's increasingly clear that something is seriously out of kilter. The journey into full-blown schizophrenia has begun.

Chapter Two

First Encounters With *Them*: Symptoms and Paranoia

My Story

After my failures in college over a period of several years, and after experiencing only limited success when I pursued a less challenging field of study, I decided that I was not meant to earn a college degree. At the time, I had a strong desire to work for myself; I'd always dreamed of being an entrepreneur of some sort. I thought I had enough drive, energy, and determination to be successful as an independent worker. I finally made the decision to strike out on my own, and to give all my time and effort to creating a career for myself. I stopped going to school and I quit my job.

Initially, I wanted to be a computer graphics specialist. I thought I could create brochures, advertisements, videos, animation, and other digital art. Maybe I could create interactive kiosks to provide local area information to hotel guests.

I bought a top-of-the-line computer and a variety of software programs, accruing several thousand dollars of credit card debt that I had no immediate way to repay. I realized quickly that I didn't have a good strategy for attracting customers and earning income. Somehow, I needed to pay off my debts, so

I started doing small handyman jobs part time. To my surprise, after about a month I had all the work I could handle as a handyman. It seemed I was finding customers for this work rather easily. I changed my mind: Instead of a computer graphics specialist, I would be a professional handyman.

A Change of Plan

In a short while, I was overwhelmed with work but I wasn't earning much money. It turns out I had a lot to learn about business. Being inexperienced, I wasn't good at estimating how long jobs would take, and I often greatly underestimated the amount of labor required for a particular task. For instance, I might estimate that a job would take two hours, when in fact it took me four. I also underestimated the cost of materials. When I expected to earn 20 dollars an hour, I often ended up earning only five.

Another problem was lack of tools. Almost every new job required some tool that I didn't own. In the beginning, I was purchasing new tools all the time, and the combination of poor estimating and investment in new tools was crippling me financially. Some days, I earned only 20 or 30 dollars. After paying for food, gas, and insurance, I was left with nothing. I wasn't paying anything on my debts, and the interest on them was snowballing.

It was the fall of 1995 and I was 24 years old. I was working hard to attract new customers and to keep the ones I already had. I desperately wanted to project an image of competence, quality, and value to my customers, but I gradually started to develop anxieties about my workmanship. I was obsessive about making everything look

I worried constantly about what my customers thought of me.

perfect and completing jobs in a reasonable amount of time. I worried constantly about what my customers thought of me. "Did I do that job well enough? Could I do it better next time? Am I being productive?" These were thoughts that occurred to me constantly. My worrying only distracted me from my work. In many cases, obsessive thinking probably caused me to be less productive and make more mistakes.

Being Watched

About this time, the tide of paranoia started to rise slowly in my brain. I was experiencing some performance anxiety, but this anxiety was combined with paranoid feelings. I became more self-conscious, and wondered whether people were watching me while I was working—especially my customers. My paranoid thoughts often related to my work: If I made a mistake, or if I did something I thought was inefficient, I would think "Did my customer see me make that mistake? Maybe they think I'm not a good worker. Are they watching me now?"

The paranoia started mildly. Although I often *wondered* whether my customers were watching me, I did not *believe* they were really doing it. Instead I wondered if they *might* be watching me, a thought that caused a great deal of anxiety, and this uncertainty was much more disturbing than actual surveillance. Strangely, if a customer stood behind me and watched every single thing I did, I would feel little or no anxiety. It was when I wasn't sure if they were watching me or not that I experienced the most anxiety of all.

I always wanted to do the best job in the fastest and most efficient way possible. But when I first started as a handyman I made a lot of mistakes, and although I could correct most of them, they still bothered me greatly. I often felt inadequate and incompetent, and every error I made reinforced the idea that

I wasn't a good handyman, making me worry that my customers would notice my failings. I often felt the urge to look over my shoulder to see if they were watching. At the age of 25, these thoughts started to occur to me quite often, maybe as much as a dozen times a day.

As the months passed, my skills as a handyman improved immensely, but I remained very critical of myself, and I lacked confidence. The paranoid thoughts increased in frequency and intensity, and after two years, I found myself wondering hundreds of times a day whether I was being watched. These thoughts expanded beyond my customers, too. I also wondered whether the neighbors were watching, or somebody else. When I went to the mall, or a large store, I wondered whether the security guards were watching me. I became very sensitive to security cameras, especially in large megastores, banks, and convenience stores. They often made me think I was being watched exclusively. As more time passed, I started to get a general feeling that I was being observed wherever I went, by the general public. I felt exposed and self-conscious in every public place—like I was on display at a zoo.

About this time I met Dan and Helen, an affluent married couple who quickly became my best customers. They had a large house and several acres of property, which they maintained in excellent condition. They always had work for me to do, and after a few months, we developed a great rapport. They liked the work I did for them, and they liked me. I became very fond of them and developed a deep respect for their opinion and judgment. They occasionally invited me to join them for lunch or dinner.

Throughout the following year, my anxieties and the obsessive thoughts associated with them continued to plague me. At one point, I decided to go to a psychiatrist. I had only one meeting with him. I explained that I was having anxieties about my work performance. I didn't tell him that I wondered whether people were watching me or not, because I didn't really believe that they were—it was just a strong suspicion. I did know for a fact that I had a lot of performance anxiety, so this was all I mentioned to the doctor. I realize now that this was a mistake. If I had related my paranoia to him at this point, I might have spared myself some of the unpleasant effects of schizophrenia that I would soon be experiencing. If you ever visit a psychiatrist yourself, I encourage you to explain everything that you are thinking about, whether you know it to be true or not. The job of a psychiatrist is to assess your mental status in general, not to validate what you already know is true. In my case, the psychiatrist merely confirmed that I was having an excessive level of anxiety, and he suggested that I try an anti-anxiety medication. I told him I would consider medication for the future, but ultimately I decided against it. I thought my anxiety was a result of poor performance, and I couldn't see how a medication would make me perform better—so why should I take it? I now understand that if I had taken the medication, I might have been better able to concentrate on my work, instead of obsessing about it.

If you ever visit a psychiatrist yourself, I encourage you to explain everything that you are thinking about, whether you know it to be true or not.

A New Opportunity

At about the age of 27, I ran into an old acquaintance who mentioned that he might have an opening for a part-time handyman where he was currently working. The job would pay about 30% more than I was earning. He gave me his business card and about a month later we arranged a meeting at his office. When I saw the building he worked in, I knew it was a good opportunity for me.

John Carmichael worked for a telecommunications giant on a project that would provide voice and data communications via satellite to any location on earth. A person with a special satellite phone would be able to communicate from anywhere on the surface of the earth, including anywhere on the oceans, or at the north and south poles. The design of the network included about 70 satellites and half a dozen earth stations located at various positions all over the globe. The facility where John worked was the main nerve center of the entire network. I estimated that a lot of money was spent to construct the building, and that the company would be willing to spend a lot of money to maintain it. John explained that the facility needed a part-time worker to take care of things like replacing light bulbs, painting, wall repair, and other maintenance needs. I submitted a proposal for my services and, after a few months, it was accepted. I was elated.

I was looking forward to working at the facility, but there was one major problem: It was a high-security building. There were cameras in every room, every hallway, and all over the exterior of the building. I did not anticipate how this environment would affect me.

I began working at the facility in February of 1998. From the first day I felt the strain of the cameras bearing down on me. I couldn't escape the idea that I was being watched all the time. The feeling that I was under observation was permanently burned into my brain. When the day ended and I left the building, I felt that somehow I was still being watched. Before, I had felt that people in general were watching me. Now, the feeling was associated specifically with this new facility. As the months passed, the feelings of anxiety grew stronger, along with my suspicions. I knew that no single person would have the ability to watch me all the time, so I thought "THEY are watching me, collectively."

I never recognized that I had been experiencing the same type of paranoid feelings over a period of several years. I didn't realize that the paranoid anxiety I experienced at the facility was the same anxiety I felt while working elsewhere. The feelings were overpowering—affecting my reason, thinking, judgment, and perception of the world. I didn't realize that the feelings were abnormal and unusual.

I began to believe that the facility would be of great interest to the U.S. government, especially the defense industry and the intelligence community. I expected the Defense Department would be their largest customer, and because of this I thought the facility might be under severe scrutiny. I had been given master keys and access to virtually every room in the building, so I thought perhaps I was being spied on for this reason. In my mind, somehow the facility, the Defense Department, and the intelligence community were all related—they were working together.

Because of the turmoil in my mind, I couldn't work effectively on any task. A job that should take 10 minutes to complete was taking me 30 minutes. I couldn't continue this way and still expect to perform well. I tried very hard to focus on my duties and to tune out any thoughts that weren't directly related to the job I was doing. But I just couldn't do it. The thoughts continued to plague me—every day, every week, every month. They were unstoppable, and they would only get worse.

Some coincidences that took place in my personal life further convinced me that people were spying on me. I started having problems with my home computer, problems that usually happened when I was connected to the Internet. Letters would appear that I did not type, or the cursor would move when I was not moving the mouse. My system would crash often. I wondered if someone had remote control of my computer, and if so, whether they could intercept everything I was doing. In reality, I probably had a computer virus, but I suspected the intelligence community (and indirectly, the facility) was the culprit.

One night I was driving home and decided to take a dirt road that was seldom used. I had never seen anyone turn onto this road. I soon noticed that a van was behind me. After several miles, the dirt road turned back onto the main road, but the van was still behind me. Why had it taken the same road? Maybe it was following me. What was the truth?

I imagined that the van behind me was driven by a private investigator hired by people at the facility to follow me. I became very distraught by this thought. I thought I was becoming a problem for them. Perhaps my behavior at work made them unsure of my mental status. Perhaps they had hired a private investigator to observe my behavior outside of work.

An Unanswered Message

I wanted to take some action to alleviate my fears. I wanted to let the people at the facility know that I wasn't going to be a problem for them. I decided to send a message to that effect through my personal computer. If what I suspected was true, the people at the facility would get the message—but if none of it was true, no harm would be done. I typed the message and sent it to my own e-mail address. I hoped that the intelligence community would intercept this message and provide it to the people at the facility.

The next time I went into work, I noticed some things that seemed peculiar to me. I usually saw security guards walking around all day long, but this day, I didn't see them at all. When I looked at the security cameras, it seemed they were never pointed at me. I wondered if THEY had received my message. They were trying not to make me nervous. Perhaps.

I wondered if THEY had received my message.

Shortly afterward, the facility hired a new manager named Bill. I was immediately suspicious of him and thought he might have been hired to deal specifically with me. But over the next several months, I became very fond of him. He was a hard worker and genuinely cared for people, providing guidance and assistance wherever possible to those who worked for him. Of the 20 or so managers or bosses I have had in my life, Bill was the best. Later, when my illness was severe, I put Bill in a difficult situation, treated him unfairly, and said awful things to him. I regret that. He didn't deserve it.

While I was working at the facility, I continued working for Helen and Dan several days per week. Sometime in the fall or winter, I agreed to program a computer application for Dan to keep track of his investments. Because I could only work on this project in my spare time, I explained that he would have to be patient for the results. I didn't know how long it would take. In February, I started teaching myself Windows/Database development.

Around this time, I developed another symptom of paranoia—the idea that people were talking about me. At work, at the mall, at the bank, wherever I was, I often overheard conversations between strangers. No matter what they were

Somehow their conversations seemed to have a special meaning related to me or my work.

talking about, I frequently wondered if their discussion was about me. Somehow their conversations seemed to have a special meaning related to me or my work.

In late spring or early summer, I was shopping at a large home improvement store a few miles from the facility. A man was browsing near me, and I became suspicious of him. I started talking to him, mentioning my handyman service. He told me that he ran a business himself, and seemed very interested in my work at the facility. I gave him my business card—he did not give me his.

A few weeks later, he called and offered me an opportunity working with his company. He said he did business with the CIA and FBI.

"Thanks for the offer," I told him, "but I'm happy working for myself right now."

I dismissed him too quickly. I should have investigated the opportunity, but I never got the chance. He never called back. Later, I started to wonder whether the CIA was investigating me. Were they collaborating with the facility? Was the FBI involved in some way? How could I find out the truth?

Too Many Coincidences

By now it was June. Dan and Helen had left for their summer home out of town. They had left me with the keys to their house, and permission to work there whenever I wanted. Dan had a large octagonal office in the basement, and I often used his office computer to work on his mutual fund–programming project. I was sitting at his computer late one night when I became very suspicious that someone was watching me. I looked over my shoulder and around the room. I quickly focused on a vent on one wall of the office. Because of the un-usual shape of Dan's office, and its orientation to the adjoin-ing rooms, there was some void space behind the wall, enough for a person to be hiding there. I wondered if someone was watching me through the vent. I started to wonder if Dan and Helen were somehow collaborating with the surveillance team. Were my good friends spying on me, too?

How could I find out the truth? I didn't feel that I had the right to go looking through their things. On the other hand, I didn't think there would be any harm in looking at things that were in plain sight. I started to look around the room for clues, and almost immediately found something that caught my at-tention. A plaque on Dan's bookshelf had the names of several people engraved on it. One of them stood out. *Carmichael.* Dan knew someone with the last name of Carmichael, which was not a common name. Did Dan know my friend John Carmichael, from the facility? Could they both be involved with the surveillance somehow? Until then, I had never associ-ated John Carmichael with THEM. How were Dan and John involved in this?

Often, when I was ill, my mind made connections be-tween people, places, things, and thoughts when there really *I saw a correlation between* were no relationships between *things where none existed.* them at all. I saw a correlation between things where none existed. This is a marker of schizophrenic thinking.

In August of 1999, I suddenly started to become psychotic. I am using the word *psychotic* to mean that my perception of the real world diverged sharply from reality. Although I had been having delusional thinking for many years, my illness was markedly more severe in August. Prior to this time, I had not told anyone else that I thought I was being followed, spied on, or investigated. Soon, however, my friends and family would become aware that I was having mental problems.

One Sunday night, I came home late, and I noticed a car in my neighborhood that seemed suspicious. It was moving very slowly along the road toward me without its headlights turned on. I thought, "It's Them!" I got into my truck and drove toward the car. Suddenly, it sped off. I followed it out of my neighborhood and copied down its license plate number. I immediately called the police. A few minutes later, an officer arrived and I explained what had happened. He called someone on his radio and had them check the license plate number. "That number doesn't exist in the State of Maryland," he said. I was sure I had the right number, but I wasn't sure what state the plate was from. The officer left.

I returned to my apartment and got on the Internet to try to find a Web site where I could search for license plate numbers myself. The only sites I found required a credit card payment to access any information. I gave up looking. Instead, I started to surf the Internet at random. I was highly agitated. I clicked on a link to a certain page, but instead I was redirected to a page that was blank, with no data. I went surfing in another location and clicked on a different link but was redirected again to the same blank page. I thought that was strange. I then tried to access my Internet history and attempted to connect to a Web site that I was familiar with, but once again I was redirected to the same blank page. At this point, I became convinced that my computer had been hacked. Previously, I had a little bit of doubt, but now I was 100% sure. Why else was I getting redirected to this page?

I quickly became convinced that the FBI had hacked my computer, and they were somehow working with the facility to keep me under surveillance. I certainly didn't have any real evidence to support this conclusion, but evidence isn't required for a delusion. When I was ill, my mind invented stories about the world, and I was predisposed to believing these stories were true, no matter how unlikely or outrageous they were. Sometimes I knew I had no proof, but my mind tried to rationalize my beliefs by inventing additional stories that made the beliefs seem more plausible.

> *I certainly didn't have any real evidence to support this conclusion, but evidence isn't required for a delusion.*

I was so sure that the FBI had hacked my computer that I immediately called my dad and a close friend and asked them to come to my apartment. It was almost midnight, but they arrived within minutes. I explained to them that I thought the FBI had planted something on my computer system and was monitoring my online activities. I asked them for their advice, but they had none to offer.

On Tuesday, I was back at work at the facility. As usual, Bill had a list of things for me to do. One of them involved some modifications to be made to a cubicle in the building. While I was working on this, the employee who occupied the cubicle came along. I explained the modifications, but he had different ideas about what should be done. I decided to talk to Bill first before making any unplanned changes. I immediately went to look for him.

"How is the work going?" he asked. I explained what had happened—that the employee wanted me to do something different. He seemed to become very angry with me. "Listen. When I give you something to do, I want you to do it my way! I don't care what anybody else says! Do what I tell you to do!"

Bill had never reacted like this before. He had never repri-manded me for anything. I felt like he was yelling at me, or scolding me. I became very upset and started to cry uncon-trollably. Bill said, "Hey, come on now, stop this. Pull yourself together. Calm down now." But I couldn't stop. He said very little to me the rest of the day.

The next day, I decided to take my computer to a store to have the hard drive copied. I was sure that the FBI had planted spyware on my computer and I wanted to preserve the evidence in case something happened. I thought what they had done was illegal and I wanted to expose them. My plan was to take the copied hard drive to a computer security expert and have the contents examined.

On the drive to the store, I stopped at a traffic light. While I was stopped, the automatic locks on the doors of the van suddenly unlocked. I pushed the button to lock the doors. Immediately they unlocked again. I thought, "That's strange." I pushed the lock button a second time. Once again, all the doors unlocked. I held my finger on the lock button for 20 seconds. As soon as I released it, they unlocked. As I sat there thinking about the problem, the doors locked themselves, then unlocked, several times in a row.

Maybe this was a hallucination, but it seemed real to me. I thought, "It's THEM! They're trying to freak me out!" I had intense anxiety. I became afraid that the FBI would pull up alongside the van, unlock the doors, and steal my computer, with all the evidence on it. I was now sure that I was right—they had been following me around 24 hours a day. Only two blocks away was the office of a lawyer I knew, and I thought maybe he could help. I arrived at his office within a minute and I carried my computer in with me. I explained that I thought the FBI had planted software on my computer and was tracking my activities illegally. I asked if he would be willing to take possession of my computer. I thought it would be safer in his office. He suggested that I contact the local police instead.

I was afraid to drive to the police station by myself, so I called a friend and asked him to meet me at the lawyer's office. When he arrived, I told him the same thing I told the lawyer, and he agreed to follow me to the closest city police station. Once there, an officer came out to talk to me, and my friend said to him, "This man here needs your help. Please listen to him. He is not crazy!"

At this point, most of my family and friends were not yet fully aware that I was having mental problems. They actually believed that I might be in trouble with the FBI. Because they hadn't noticed any previous psychological problems, they tended to believe what I told them. Soon, they would begin to realize the truth.

> *...most of my family and friends were not yet fully aware that I was having mental problems.*

Later that night, I was thinking about the day's events. Why did they operate my door locks like that? I thought back to one of my theories about the surveillance. Perhaps they actually wanted to hire me for a special job, and needed to know how I would react under stress. Perhaps Bill had been testing me the other day when he scolded me.

I thought back to the telephone call I received from the man I'd met at the home improvement store, asking if I wanted to work for his company at the CIA or FBI. Maybe he was with the surveillance team. Perhaps they just wanted to see what I would say about working there? Maybe this job is super secret—the type of job that no one except me and them will ever know about. So secret that they don't conduct the usual background checks, talking to your family and friends, because they don't want anyone to know about it. Instead, they keep you under surveillance for years before even offering you the job. Maybe, I thought, that's what's happening to me. Maybe all this surveillance is a necessary part of the hiring process. Maybe Bill was a CIA agent assigned to work on my case. I decided that I could no longer work at the facility without knowing the truth.

Uncertain Assumptions

On Thursday morning, I called Bill and told him I could no longer work at the facility. "Why not?" I made up an excuse, saying, "I have a conflict of interest." I arranged to pick up my things at one o'clock. He didn't ask me any other questions.

Next I called Dan and asked if he would meet with me that morning. At that point, I still trusted him. I told him I thought my computer had been hacked and that the facility was involved in some way. He agreed that if I was not comfortable working there, I should quit. "Just be aware of what assumptions you're making," he said.

I arrived at the facility in the afternoon. My dad went along with me. Bill met us at the main entrance. "Kurt, I don't know what assumptions you are making, but if you ever want to come back here, just call me . . . you can come back any time." I was suspicious. Bill mentioned making assumptions, and so had Dan. Did they know something I didn't?

On the way home, my dad and I stopped at a golf range to drive some balls. I thought the people around me were part of the surveillance team, even though most of them had arrived before me. I saw a group of people sitting at a picnic table, talking about their work, but I started to believe they were talking about me. While I was sitting on a bench, a large bug fluttered by and landed on a bush, which led me to think about hidden microphones being called "bugs" and about insects being called "bugs." I began to believe that this bug was a surveillance device designed by the CIA to look like a real insect.

I stayed in my apartment for most of the next day. My imagination was running wild. I was thinking about how computer systems had become more powerful and more sophisticated over the last 50 years. What impossible tasks would become possible in the future thanks to computer technology? I wondered if computers would be able to send data directly to the brain by some type of neural connection. Could such a computer generate a virtual reality? Maybe I was hooked up to one of these machines right now! Maybe my whole world was actually generated by a virtual reality machine connected to my brain! How would I know whether this was true or not?

I began to hear clicking noises. They weren't coming from the real world, but they didn't seem to be in my imagination either. These noises seemed to be coming from some place outside the universe, from somewhere I had never perceived before. I thought, "Maybe I am actually in a virtual reality. Maybe these noises are coming from the real world." I wondered if I was really human. "Maybe I'm not human at all. Maybe I'm some type of alien, connected to a virtual reality machine run by aliens with advanced technology. Maybe I'm in some type of laboratory."

I began to feel despair, fear, and anxiety at the prospect of discovering that everything I had ever known was not real. I didn't want to know the truth. I didn't want to wake up from the dream. I began to think that I needed to have faith that the universe I knew actually existed. "I must believe my life to exist. To have meaning, I have to have faith in that." In a few minutes, the clicking noises stopped, along with my out-of-body experience.

The next day I woke up with chills. I did not remember going to bed. I had never had a loss of memory in my entire life. I looked at the thermometer on the wall: 73 degrees. There was no reason why I should have the chills. I seemed to recall that chills could be a side effect of anesthesia. I tried to remember the night before, but couldn't remember anything. I thought, "I really had strange thoughts last night. THEY must have given me some kind of hallucinogenic drugs. Then, they gave me an amnesiac. Why would they do that? Maybe they abducted me and gave me some kind of truth serum. Maybe they interviewed me."

Later that day, I decided to go visit my brother and his family, and ended up spending the night. The next morning, my sister-in-law invited me to go with them to church, but I recall that I said something rude to her and she left abruptly. As I was driving home, I started to think about religion, and to have grandiose feelings. I thought I was involved in something huge. I felt like I was joined with the universe on some metaphysical, philosophical, and spiritual level. I wondered if God was somehow controlling the direction of my life for some grand purpose that would affect us all. I thought for a few seconds that maybe I was Jesus. Then, I realized that I didn't believe in the divinity of Jesus. Then I thought "Maybe that's what THEY think. Maybe they think I'm Jesus."

I started to believe that there were many agents following me that day. Perhaps 50 or 100 of them. I thought, "Why would there be so many people following me?" I had to talk to someone who knew more than I did. I thought Bill might be one of those people. I had suspected he was working for THEM, but I trusted him anyway.

I was sure Bill was somewhere in the facility, even though it was Sunday, so I drove there to look for him. When I couldn't find him, I told the security guard on duty to page him with a text message. "What should I say?" he asked. I told him to say, "Tell him it's his last chance." What I meant was, "This is your last chance to talk to me." The guard said, "Are you sure you want to say that?" "Yes."

I waited ten minutes for Bill to respond, but he never did. The guard asked me what I wanted to do. I said, "Ok, I guess I'll be leaving then."

"I can't let you do that." What? What did he mean? Was he joking? I didn't think so. He was standing between me and the door leading out to my truck. I didn't trust them. What were they going to do with me? I quickly decided to leave my truck behind and exited through a different door. I walked out quickly without looking back. The guard did not follow me.

An Imagination Run Wild

I walked about half a mile to a nearby hospital, where I called a taxi. My plan was to take public transportation back to Maryland, and call my folks to come pick me up. I was highly agitated at this point. I was suspicious of everyone, everywhere. When the taxi arrived, I gave the driver very specific instructions—I was even suspicious of him. He drove about five miles, then suddenly turned off the route I had given him. "Where are you going?" I asked. "I know a shortcut," he said. I thought, "He must be with Them! He's kidnapping me! What are They going to do with me?" I asked, "Are you going to kill me?" I didn't wait to find out what would happen—I bailed out of the cab at the next stoplight.

I was about six to ten miles from the facility. I thought I could walk to the airport, where I knew I could catch a bus to the nearest train station. I started walking along the highway, but after a few minutes, I noticed a white SUV driving alongside me. It stopped, and a man got out. It was Bill. He was yelling at me. "Kurt! Wait! I want to talk to you!"

I thought Bill must definitely be with Them. He must have followed me there, and I no longer trusted him. I turned toward him and spewed a short barrage of profanity, then turned in the other direction and started to run away. I found I couldn't run that well, because I was wearing floppy boat shoes. I took them off and started to run barefoot. Bill followed me in his vehicle and I started to hear sirens behind me. He must have called the police.

The police questioned me for a few minutes. They wanted to know why I was running along the highway, and why I had left my truck at the facility. I don't know exactly what I said to them, but I somehow convinced them to take me to the airport a few miles away. Once there, I caught a bus to the metro station.

I suspected there were several agents with me on the bus. When it stopped, I waited for everyone else to get off, and I carefully watched where they went. On the metro platform, instead of getting on the first train, I waited for the next one, wanting to lose the agents. I only took the train a few stops, and got off. I was still sure I was being followed, even though I didn't see anyone following me. I walked around at random, trying to confuse the agents.

I was still sure I was being followed, even though I didn't see anyone following me.

I went into a nearby restaurant and ordered something to eat. I started to believe there were agents all over the restaurant, including the people I saw with children. Afterward I walked

to the next train stop, over a mile away. I was trying to rationalize why there would be hundreds of agents following me.
I couldn't. But I never disbelieved it.

Eventually, I made it to the train station in Maryland, and
I called my parents to come pick me up. When they arrived,
I discovered that they had spoken to Bill on the phone. They
said very little. I think they realized now that I was having
mental problems.

A few days later, my parents arranged an appointment with
a psychiatrist. At first, I didn't see him, but my family and
friends met with him. Why should I talk to a psychiatrist? How
could he influence the FBI, CIA, or the facility? At this point I
still believed that the problem was with those around me, and
not with me myself. Later, I did meet with the psychiatrist, but
I told him nothing. Based on the testimony of my friends and
family, he diagnosed me with bipolar disorder and prescribed
Lithium. I never took it regularly.

I started to believe that maybe I was part of some long-term
project. Maybe They had been following me for much longer
than I suspected. I thought about frequent nightmares I used
to have when I was a teenager. Maybe They had abducted me
when I was a teenager, and had brainwashed me. My imagination was running wild.

I imagined that I was in a conflict with the CIA. I thought
there were two groups of CIA agents. One group, the "Bad"
agents, was planning to kill me. These are the agents that had
tried to abduct me, that had drugged me, that had used psychological warfare on me. I imagined that the "Bad" agents
might be killing everyone who knew anything about the project. The other group, the "Good" agents, was trying to keep
me safe. I thought perhaps some of the "Good" agents might
have believed (erroneously) that I was Jesus.

I knew that I was behaving strangely. I thought this was due to the brainwashing process. I thought that They had brainwashed me to become a "super-agent." The brainwashing had planted subconscious thoughts that would make me more sensitive to surveillance. These thoughts enabled me to detect when anyone was following me, or observing me. This was the reason I became so anxious when They started following me. Subconsciously, I was able to detect Them.

It was with all these thoughts in mind that I crafted a long, rambling e-mail describing the various delusions and conspiracy theories I'd come to believe over the past several months, and how I was not a threat to the FBI, CIA, or the facility. I believed they would intercept it, and hoped it would end the surveillance. I emailed it to myself, but my mother was able to get a copy. After reading it, I'm sure there was no doubt left in her mind that I was having mental problems.

My parents soon became reluctant to let me go anywhere by myself. I'd quit my job at the facility, and I was not working as a handyman anymore. I was never leaving the house. In a few weeks, the most severe symptoms of schizophrenia had decreased in intensity, probably due to decreased stress levels. I started to work more aggressively on Dan's mutual fund application. By the end of December, I had completed it successfully. Nothing abnormal or unusual happened for the next several months.

The Big Picture

At its core, schizophrenia is a disorder of perception. The sights, sounds, and experiences perceived by a person with schizophrenia seem just as "real" as those experienced by anyone else. Yet the reality of schizophrenia is very different from reality as perceived by most people. When you're listening to the radio in a healthy frame of mind, you might hear your favorite song or the afternoon traffic report—but when you're having a schizophrenic episode, you might hear a voice issuing warnings directly to you.

The behavior of a person with schizophrenia often seems inexplicable to outside observers. But to the person who is ill, it makes complete sense in the context of his or her reality. Imagine yourself walking alone into a dimly lit apartment. In a corner, you glimpse a shadowy shape that looks like a man, and your heart leaps into your throat. Perhaps an intruder is hiding in the corner, waiting to attack you. On closer inspection, though, you realize that the shape is actually just a coat hanging there. You quickly realize your error and revise your interpretation of how threatening the situation is. But when you have schizophrenia, errors of perception and interpretation aren't always corrected, and the way you think and behave reflects these distorted views.

What Are Positive and Negative Symptoms of Schizophrenia?

The symptoms of schizophrenia come in two basic varieties: positive and negative. Positive symptoms include the abnormal perceptions, thoughts, and behaviors that are *produced by* the disease. These symptoms represent the type of break with reality that many people associate with severe mental illness. Psychosis is another term that's used for the positive symptoms of schizophrenia, while the loss of contact with reality is sometimes referred to as a psychotic break. Positive symptoms may wax and wane, and at times, they may be barely noticeable to others. But when such symptoms are severe, they can lead to behavior that is dramatically unusual.

Negative symptoms, in contrast, include normal emotions and behaviors that are *reduced by* schizophrenia. Such symptoms often involve a gradual withdrawal from the world and loss of interest in caring for oneself. While negative symptoms are less dramatic than positive ones, they can create at least as much chaos in the person's daily life and family relationships. It isn't easy to live with or care for someone who offers total indifference in return. In addition, it's not uncommon for others to misinterpret negative symptoms as signs of coldness or laziness. Below, we'll take a closer look at both positive and negative symptoms of schizophrenia.

POSITIVE SYMPTOMS

- *Delusions* are false personal beliefs that have no basis in reality and remain unchanged even when the person is presented with strong evidence to the contrary. For example, a delusional person might believe that a neighbor is planting thoughts in his mind, that a newspaper headline is directed specifically to him, or that he is actually a famous figure from history. The most common beliefs of this type are delusions of persecution, in which the person irrationally believes that he is being plotted against, spied upon, followed, tricked, or harassed.
- *Hallucinations* are false sensory impressions. The person sees, hears, smells, tastes, or feels something that isn't really there. Auditory hallucinations, in which the person hears things that no one else can hear, are by far the most common type. They usually take the form of

"hearing voices," which may warn of danger, comment on the person's behavior, or command the person to do things. Some people with schizophrenia hear voices for a long time before the disease reaches the point where other people notice that something is wrong.

Illness or Individuality?

The world would be an infinitely more boring place if we all saw things exactly the same way. Fortunately, that's far from the case. There are plenty of perfectly healthy, rational people who firmly believe in government conspiracies, alien abductions, or out-of-body experiences. They may be convinced that they've seen a ghost or heard the voice of God. Does this mean they're mentally ill? Not necessarily. To one degree or another, we've all probably held some beliefs that were out of the ordinary, but that doesn't automatically mean they're unhealthy.

No single belief or behavior, no matter how eccentric, is enough in itself to identify someone as having schizophrenia. To qualify as schizophrenia, other criteria must be met as well:

- The symptoms must interfere with a person's social relationships, ability to take care of himself or herself, or capacity to function at school or work. Without such dysfunction, there's no disorder.
- The most severe symptoms must last for at least a month, unless that period is cut short by successful treatment.
- The symptoms aren't explained by substance abuse, another medical condition, or the side effects of a medication.

- *Disorganized thoughts and speech* involve an inability to organize thoughts, connect them logically, and express them coherently. The disordered thoughts and speech that result are prominent symptoms of schizophrenia— some would say the *most* prominent ones. In some cases, the person's thoughts may frequently slip off track or jump unpredictably from topic to topic. In other cases, the person may stop speaking abruptly in mid-thought, respond to questions with answers that are unrelated, or make up unintelligible words. At times, the person's speech may become so garbled that it's nearly incomprehensible to other people.

- *Disorganized behavior* is an extension of disorganized thinking. Some people with schizophrenia have trouble accomplishing even the most basic goals, such as practicing good personal hygiene or preparing their own meals. They may look disheveled or dress in a bizarre fashion. Others may behave in a childlike manner or become agitated for no obvious reason.

- *Catatonic behavior* involves a marked decrease in a person's responsiveness to the outside world, as shown by severe disturbances in movement. The person may become immobile, resist efforts to be moved, or seem to get stuck in a bizarre posture. In other cases, the person may engage in incessant, purposeless movements. Catatonic behavior was more common in the days before effective treatments were available. Thankfully, it is relatively rare today.

Other Faces of Schizophrenia: "Steve"

Steve was an art student in his senior year at college when the first psychotic episode struck. In hindsight, he thinks the earliest warning sign was increased conflict with others. "I hadn't been in too many arguments before, but suddenly I was getting into arguments all the time. Someone else would say something, and I was sure it was offensive or untrue. It's only looking back that I realize that what people actually said was different from what I thought they said."

Over time, Steve's behavior grew more erratic. "I was walking the street at all hours of the night downtown, going places that were dangerous," he says. "Hanging out in parks and such at odd hours—I didn't realize how dangerous it was. When I got home, I would watch television, and the people on TV were sending me signals by the way they blinked. Then strange things started happening to my body, like I stopped making eye contact because it physically hurt my eyes."

Steve continues, "One day, my sister came over to my house, and I wouldn't come out of my room." She yelled through to door to ask what was wrong, and Steve replied that he was worried he would hurt someone. "She was like, 'What are you talking about? You wouldn't hurt a fly.' And I was like, 'Well, if I look somebody in the eye, it might hurt them, because it definitely hurts me.'"

Steve's sister took him to a mental hospital, but they didn't admit him that day. His illness didn't appear to be serious enough for hospitalization based on the answers he gave to questions during an evaluation. So Steve returned home, but his condition continued to worsen. "I would sit still—absolutely, positively still for a long period of time," he recalls. "And I would think, 'Hey, I'm good for sitting still. This is something I can do that other people can't.' But it wasn't normal, and people looked at me oddly."

"It wasn't like I was ill all the time," Steve says. "I did have moments when I could see that what I was doing wasn't right. But I couldn't control going in and out of it. It just happened." A few days later, he returned to the hospital, and this time he was admitted. During his week-and-a-half stay there, Steve was diagnosed with schizophrenia, and he started taking medication to control his symptoms.

That was in 1983. Over the next 15 years, Steve went through many ups and downs as he struggled to get his illness under control. Then in 1998, he finally had a breakthrough when he found a medication that worked well for him. Around the same time, he began going to a drop-in center for people with mental health issues, where he found much-needed support from the new friends he made.

Steve now considers himself recovered. He works with mental health consumers, and he's also a busy artist. At the time of this interview, his paintings were on display in two shows in the large city where he lives. Steve believes that art has played a critical role in his improvement. "Art is problem solving," he says. "You want to communicate a message, and you also have to arrange all the elements—line, color, shape—in a pleasing composition. It keeps my mind active. Because if you just take the medicine and sit around all day watching TV, it's not going to help you as much as if you take the medicine and then use your mind."

NEGATIVE SYMPTOMS

- *Flat affect* refers to an extreme lack of any signs of emotional expression. In psych lingo, affect (pronounced "AF-fekt") is a person's changing emotional state. Most of us are constantly sending out signals about how we're feeling at any given point in time. We laugh for joy, frown with displeasure, bounce from excitement, or yell in anger. However, these signals are often greatly reduced in people with schizophrenia. Their facial expression, body language, and tone of voice may stay largely unchanged, and they may avoid making eye contact. For other people, this can be one of the most disconcerting aspects of schizophrenia.
- *Alogia* refers to a reduction in the quantity or quality of speech. In some cases, people begin speaking infrequently and responding to questions with only curt replies. In other cases, the amount of speech is normal, but the information conveyed is minimal. People may repeat themselves, make meaningless comments, or become overly literal or overly abstract in the way they talk.
- *Avolition* refers to a pervasive lack of initiative and motivation. This is more than just your garden-variety trouble getting started on a homework assignment or staying motivated to finish it. Instead, a person with schizophrenia may have trouble planning and finishing almost any task, from school to work to social activities. The person may sit for hours and have trouble mustering up enough motivation for even basic self-care activities, such as eating and bathing.

- *Anhedonia* refers to a loss of interest or pleasure in activities that a person once enjoyed. The person may abandon previous hobbies and interests as his or her world grows ever smaller and more isolated.

How Important Are Cognitive Symptoms of Schizophrenia?

Schizophrenia is also associated with cognitive symptoms that involve deficits in thinking abilities, such as making decisions, paying attention, and remembering. Because such symptoms often are subtle and can only be detected with sophisticated testing, they were relatively ignored for many years. Recently, however, scientists have come to appreciate just how disabling these symptoms can be. Examples of cognitive symptoms include problems with:

- Absorbing information, interpreting it, and making decisions based upon it
- Paying attention and shifting focus when appropriate
- Keeping recently learned information in mind and using it right away

Outside of a formal testing situation, the boundary between cognitive symptoms and negative symptoms often is blurry at best. For instance, when someone fails to finish a task, is it because of the inability to pay attention (a cognitive symptom), the lack of motivation (a negative symptom), or both? The answer to that question may not be immediately apparent. What *is* clear is that both cognitive and negative symptoms make it very hard to function in daily life. They also can be extremely frustrating and cause great emotional distress. Although they may not be as blatant as positive symptoms, they can be every bit as debilitating—perhaps even more so.

Are People With Schizophrenia Aware of How Sick They Are?

Do people with schizophrenia realize that something is terribly wrong? Some do, some don't—and the degree of insight may vary within individuals depending on how sick they are at the time. Self-awareness, when it comes, is a double-edged sword. Lack of awareness insulates a person from what's happening, and when that insulation is stripped away, the shock and fear can be intense. It may be alternately frightening and confusing to believe that you're the subject of a stealthy investigation by the CIA. But that's nothing compared to the shattering realization that it's your own mind that is tricking you and your own senses that are not to be trusted.

Once you have identified the true enemy, you can begin fighting back much more effectively.

Yet on balance, self-awareness is more blessing than curse. It's a vital ingredient in seeking help and making the most of treatment. Initially, insight may bring pain and fear, but ultimately, it brings hope. Once you have identified the true enemy, you can begin fighting back much more effectively.

What Are the Different Types of Schizophrenia?

Schizophrenia is an amazingly diverse illness. No two people experience it the same way, and even the experts have difficulty summing it up in a tidy definition. Many people have several of the symptoms described above, but some have only delusions or hallucinations that are bizarre or disabling enough to wreak havoc on their lives.

For the sake of communication, it's helpful for professionals to have a shorthand that quickly conveys the general features of an individual's schizophrenia. To this end, people with schizophrenia are sometimes grouped into categories, called subtypes. A doctor's decision about the subtype to which a given patient should be assigned is based upon that person's dominant symptoms at the time of evaluation.

Yet it's no surprise that a disorder as messy and unpredictable as schizophrenia refuses to fit neatly into prelabeled boxes. Many people actually have a mix of various types of symptoms, and these symptoms may change over time. In addition, research has shown that the classic subtypes, which are based on categories first defined in the nineteenth century, have limited value for predicting the course of a particular person's illness or the effectiveness of a specific treatment. As a result, efforts are now underway to develop more useful classification systems. In the meantime, however, you may hear these terms used to describe broad categories of schizophrenia.

SUBTYPES OF SCHIZOPHRENIA

- *Paranoid schizophrenia* is characterized by prominent delusions and/or frequent auditory hallucinations. The delusions often center on themes of persecution. People with paranoid schizophrenia may hold an unshakable belief that they are being schemed against, spied upon, lied to, or otherwise mistreated, despite the lack of any rational basis for this belief. Also common are delusions of grandeur, in which people have an irrational and highly exaggerated sense of their own power, knowledge, or special relationship to God or a famous person.

Auditory hallucinations may take the form of voices saying things that are consistent with the delusions, which further confirms the person's belief in them. The person's outward manner may reflect what's going on inside his or her head. Thus, people with delusions of persecution may seem angry or anxious, while those with delusions of grandeur may have a haughty or patronizing air.

Two Disorders in One

Schizoaffective disorder isn't a type of schizophrenia, but rather a separate disorder that's closely related. At times, a person with this two-for-one condition is bothered mainly by delusions or hallucinations just like those of someone with schizophrenia. At other times, the delusions or hallucinations are mixed with a severe disturbance in mood. When you look at the course of the illness over a long period, the mood disturbance is there for much, but not all, of the time.

The mood part of schizoaffective disorder can take the form of depression, mania, or both. Depression is a sad or low mood that gives rise to symptoms such as lack of energy, trouble concentrating, feelings of worthlessness, thoughts of death, and changes in appetite, sleep, and activity level. Mania is an overly high mood that gives rise to symptoms such as grandiose ideas, decreased need for sleep, racing thoughts, risk taking, and increased talking or activity.

Even for professionals, it isn't always easy to decide whether a person has schizophrenia, a severe mood disorder, or schizoaffective disorder. Many symptoms of schizophrenia resemble those of depression (for example, lack of energy) or mania (for example, grandiose ideas). In addition, severe depression or mania itself can cause hallucinations or delusions. The decision about which disorder to diagnose is often based on subtle differences in the timing and duration of symptoms. Not surprisingly, many people who start out with one diagnosis eventually have it changed as times goes on and more symptoms emerge.

Compared to the other subtypes, paranoid schizophrenia doesn't take as harsh a toll on thinking abilities
such as attention, memory, and planning. It tends to
start later in life and be more stable. Some evidence
suggests that the odds of recovery may be better with
paranoid schizophrenia than with the other types.

- *Disorganized schizophrenia* is characterized by disorganized speech and behavior along with flat or inappropriate affect. Although we can never know exactly
what's going on inside someone else's mind, we can
draw conclusions based upon what that person says and
does. In the case of people with disorganized schizophrenia, their speech and behavior suggest a mind in
which normal chains of association have been broken,
leaving behind only a jumble of disconnected thoughts.

  People with disorganized schizophrenia may ramble
on about nonsensical ideas, laugh at inappropriate
moments, or grimace for no apparent reason. They also
may find it nearly impossible to accomplish even the
simplest goals, such as showering, dressing, and preparing food. As a result, people with disorganized
schizophrenia may look unkempt, dress bizarrely, and
take poor care of their physical health. To other people,
the overall impression they create is often decidedly
odd.

- *Catatonic schizophrenia* is characterized by severe disturbances in movement and a marked lack of responsiveness to the outside world. Some people with
catatonic schizophrenia slide into a stupor, in which
they are immobile, mute, and completely unresponsive
to what's happening around them. Others hold
themselves in bizarre or rigid postures for hours and

resist any attempt to move them. Still others repeat the same purposeless motions over and over, or mimic another person's words or actions in a senseless, parrot-like fashion. Catatonic schizophrenia can be extremely disabling, but fortunately, it's also quite uncommon.

Schizophrenia by any name is a tough diagnosis to swallow. Even when treatment is successful, the hard truth is that most people with schizophrenia must cope with some milder residual symptoms for the rest of their days. Yet even these symptoms are manageable with proper

...the prospects for recovery will only improve in the future...

treatment and support. The good news is that many people with schizophrenia eventually go on to lead full, rewarding lives. The even better news is that the prospects for recovery will only improve in the future, as scientists keep working to develop more effective treatments for the disease.

Chapter Three

In the Grip of *Them*:
Losing Touch With Reality

My Story

After my first psychotic break in August of 1999, I stayed home most of the time. If I went out at all, it was to the coffee shop, or out for a sandwich or gelato. Other than programming Dan's mutual fund application, I did very little productive work. Because I wasn't out in public, the paranoid feelings I felt were not as intense. However, my delusions continued to be the focus of my mind. One of my theories was that the CIA wanted to recruit me for a secret job. If this wasn't true, what was I going to do for the rest of my life?

Another delusion was the one that had begun in college. Though it was less prominent in my mind, it was still strong: that I was going to discover some amazing new mathematical principle involving fractals. This had been my dream for ten years, and now I wanted to devote more time and effort to solving the fractal "riddle."

Getting Away

I decided I needed to get away from home, to take a trip, to go somewhere remote, where I could reflect on my life, meditate on mathematics, and decide my future. I had abandoned the idea that the CIA wanted to kill me. I thought if they wanted to contact me, this trip would give them the perfect opportunity. I chose to go to Glacier National Park, in Montana. I also wanted to make a stop in Chicago to visit two Italian friends working there. I purchased an open-ended rail pass, because this was the most economical way to visit both Chicago and Glacier National Park in one trip. Because I had a national rail pass, I decided I would also visit Seattle and San Francisco before returning home. I expected the trip would take two or three weeks.

As I recall, my parents didn't do much to discourage me from going on this trip. Neither did my friends. Perhaps they felt that since I was an adult, they couldn't coerce me or control me. As you will soon read, my mental problems once again intensified on this trip, and my parents had to come to my assistance. It was quite a hassle and very costly for them to arrange a flight out to Montana to rescue me. I would recommend that those with mental illnesses not travel alone unless their condition is stabilized and under control. In my case, my symptoms were milder than they had been the previous August, but they were by no means under control. I still had a full set of delusions that exposed me to a resurgence of problems.

I would recommend that those with mental illnesses not travel alone unless their condition is stabilized and under control.

It was March of 2000. I remember that I left in the afternoon from Union Station in Washington, D.C., and the train arrived in Chicago the following morning. I had very little sleep, if any. I immediately found a hotel and made arrangements to meet my Italian friends for dinner that evening. They were unaware that I had ever had any mental problems, and I don't believe they noticed anything wrong with me. Afterward, I asked them to drop me off at a bookstore a few blocks from my hotel. I purchased several books and started to walk around downtown.

Paranoia quickly set in. I was sure I was being followed. Almost everyone I saw on the street seemed to be following me. I started to walk around the city at random. Time seemed to pass very quickly. Hours seemed like minutes. I found myself nearly alone in the middle of the night. It was probably two or three o'clock in the morning, but I still wondered why I didn't see people on the street anymore. Rather than conclude that everyone was asleep at home, I concluded that no one was following anymore because they had gathered all the information they needed. Perhaps they had decided to hire me! I headed back to the hotel, thinking, "They'll be sending a representative to contact me soon."

The next morning, I boarded a train for my next stop— Grand Forks, North Dakota. I wondered when they were going to contact me.

After I had been on the train for a while, I went into the smoking car to have a cigarette. There was a girl there, and when I saw her, I thought, "This is going to be my contact." We soon started talking, and she was flirting with me the whole time. Later, we met for dinner. She was still being very forward— rubbing up against me, touching my hand, and saying very suggestive things. After dinner, she told me, "I have a bottle of wine in my cabin . . . do you want to share it with me?"

We met in her cabin a while later. We drank the whole bottle and I stayed there for an hour, maybe two, and then left. It was not the situation I anticipated. She hadn't tried to talk to me about a position with the agents who had been following me. I was confused. I got off the train early in the morning at Grand Forks.

I shared a cab ride from the train station to my hotel with a woman who handed me a religious booklet on Jesus Christ. I wondered whether she was one of the "Good" agents who thought I was Jesus. I spent a few hours reading the booklet, trying to interpret what it meant. It was propaganda implying that Jesus could change your life. I couldn't really identify with the meaning of it, but I thought I should respond to it somehow. I made notes in the margins of the booklet that expressed my opinions, and later I left the booklet somewhere I thought They would be able to retrieve it.

I spent the day wandering around Grand Forks with no destination in mind. I may have walked ten miles or more, and everywhere I went I suspected I was being followed. I went back to the hotel, and then boarded the train in the morning for Glacier National Park. While I was on the train, I tried to make sense of my beliefs. Why hadn't they contacted me? What was really going on?

I went to the dining car to have breakfast and was seated with three other strangers. I thought they were probably agents from the government, but I wanted to be sure. I believed they were spending thousands of dollars to investigate me. I thought, "What would another 15 dollars matter?" When the bill came for breakfast, I pretended that I didn't have any money. Just as I had expected, one of the gentlemen paid my bill. I took this incident to be a confirmation that everything I believed was true. They were still following me.

Glasgow, Montana

After breakfast, I became highly anxious and agitated. Why were They *still* following me? I wasn't working at the facility anymore. I tried to think of new reasons why the surveillance was still going on, but I couldn't think of any reason that really made sense. I was becoming more and more confused, disoriented, and paranoid. I started to think that people on the train were talking about me. I overheard several conversations, and somehow, no matter what they were talking about, the conversations seemed to be about me. I thought the CIA was trying to use some kind of psychological warfare techniques on me. I decided that I needed to get off the train as soon as possible.

A few minutes later, the train stopped. Where were we? I didn't know, but I had to get off, immediately. I forgot where I had left my bags. I frantically looked for them for a few minutes, but I could not locate them. If I didn't get off soon, I wouldn't get another opportunity for an hour or more. I was afraid. I needed to get off right then.

I jumped off the train and walked off the platform—without my luggage.

I didn't know where I was. I found a hotel that cost only $24 a night and learned that I was in Glasgow, Montana. I called home and left a message about where I was staying.

In the previous four days, I had had only a few hours sleep each night. I thought I should take a nap. I laid down for about an hour and tried to go to sleep, but I couldn't. Instead, I got up and decided to go out for something to eat. I went into a nearby Dairy Queen to order something and sat down. As I was eating a sandwich, a man walked in and looked in my direction. I thought, "This must be my contact." I said to him, "Have a seat!" The man was very friendly. He sat down at my table and we talked for a half an hour. I don't remember much about what we discussed. I must have been acting strangely though, because he asked me if I was autistic. I was sure he was working for the CIA, the FBI, or Congress. (After my first

psychotic episode, I had delivered a letter to several congress-
men complaining that the FBI was following me.) Why else
would he be talking to me?

I headed back to the hotel. When I arrived at my hotel
room, sitting on the dresser I found an excerpt from a letter
I had written over ten years ago
to the girl I had met in Italy.
This was certainly a hallucination, but it seemed absolutely
real. I had not been thinking
about Italy, girls, or anything remotely related to this letter.
I crumpled it up and threw it in the trash. I tried for several hours to understand how this letter was related to the
surveillance—as I had assumed it was. Was the girl I knew in
the CIA? Were people following me *more than ten years ago*?
Who had left the letter in my room? Why was it only an
excerpt of the letter? What was important about the excerpt?

I tried to review everything that had happened to me over the
past several years, with a focus on what had happened most
recently. I started to think about my experience in Chicago. I
realized that although I had *thought* people were following
me in Chicago, I did not actually have any evidence, nor did
I actually see anything that would support this conclusion. I
thought, "My God, something is wrong with my mind!" This
idea did not make me question all my delusions—just my
experience for that one day. I didn't disbelieve my delusions
because they had been present in my mind for such a long time.
They were very strongly held beliefs. This was the only time
during my illness that I thought something was wrong with my
mind. I became very scared. "Maybe I have a brain tumor!"

I went to the local medical center and demanded to have a
CAT scan. The woman on duty there must have recognized

that I was having mental problems. She asked me, "Do you have any intention of hurting yourself or someone else?" "What? Of course not! No!" She suggested that I come back the next day to talk to a doctor. I went back to the hotel.

In the lobby, I got a Coke from a vending machine and took a swig. God! It was awful! It tasted bitter. I wondered if the Coke had been poisoned. Could They have poisoned the Coke? Could They have replaced the Coke in the vending machine?

I went outside and started to wander around town. There was no one on the street and I began to believe the town was deserted. The idea that the town was deserted overpowered the more rational thought that everyone was in bed, since it was getting late. I wondered if the CIA had evacuated the town. At about this point, I started to have another hallucination. I began to hear a sound that was like car horns blaring. They sounded like they were somewhere in the distance. Dozens of cars blaring their horns. They continued to sound for at least ten minutes. I started walking in the direction of the sound to see what was going on. I had no idea where I was going.

Intrusion

I eventually came to the end of the road I was walking on. A cat came up to me and nuzzled my leg, but when I reached down to pet it, it hissed and clawed my hand. I looked at my hand and there seemed to be something very small stuck in it where the cat had scratched me. I immediately thought, "They tricked me. This cat must have been trained to attack me! What is in my hand? It must be a poison dart! The bad CIA agents are trying to kill me! I have to get this thing out of my hand, right now!" I discovered that I was standing in front of a house with a garage door that was wide open. I ran into the garage where there was an entrance to the house, which was unlocked. I was frantic. I felt I had to get the dart out of my hand right away. I thought, "Nobody is home. They have evacuated the town. I'll just go inside and find something to get this thing out." I opened the door and right in front of me was the kitchen. I started to look through the drawers to find a sharp knife. I didn't immediately find anything useful, so I decided to find the bathroom and look for some fingernail clippers that I could use to cut the dart out of my hand. I ran through the living room and went into the first bathroom I saw. There was a door through the bathroom to an adjacent bedroom. Two people were lying in bed and one of them, a man, sat up and said, "Who are you? What are you doing in our house?" I was surprised that there was anyone home. I said, "I'm sorry, I didn't think you were home. I'll leave right away." I turned and started to walk out.

The man jumped out of bed and followed me into the living room.

He said, "Wait! What are you doing in our house?"

I said, "I'm trying to find some nail clippers. I didn't think you were home. I'll leave right away."

"Wait. Who are you?"

I told him my name, and that I lived near Washington, DC.

"What are you doing here?"

"I came out here on vacation."

"What are you doing in our house?"

"I need some nail clippers . . . do you have any nail clippers? I need to get this out of my hand." By now, the woman had come out into the living room where we were standing.

"What's wrong with your hand?"

"I've got something stuck in it. I need to get it out right away. Do you have any nail clippers? Please get me some nail clippers!"

He said, "What about some tweezers? Do you want some tweezers?"

I thought the poison had already gotten into my hand. I needed some nail clippers to cut out the affected part. I said, "No. I need some nail clippers. Do you have any?"

He said to his wife, "Can you get a pair of nail clippers?" She came out a moment later with some nail clippers and handed them to me. I looked at my hand. I didn't see anything stuck in there anymore, but I thought, "Surely the poison is in my hand." I cut a piece of flesh out of my hand where I thought the dart had been.

I said, "Thanks. I'll be going now." The man said, "Wait. Where are you going to go? What are you doing here in Glasgow?" I said, "I don't know. There was some kind of intelligence problem. I got off the train." He said, "What kind of intelligence problem?" "I don't know! That's the problem!" I sat down and started to cry uncontrollably. As I was sitting there, I was still wondering why they were home. Why hadn't they been evacuated? Maybe they were CIA agents. Maybe they were with the good agents who were trying to protect me.

The man said, "Just calm down. Sit here for a moment. We're going to get you some help. Just stay here for a few moments. I'm going to call someone to come help. Is that okay?" "Yeah." I waited there for a while, crying.

He said, "Everything's going to be okay. We're getting you some help. Would you like something to drink?"

A few minutes later, a police officer arrived. He was very gentle. He talked with the man of the house for a few moments. Then he said, "I'm going to take you to the medical center." We went out to his car and drove to the medical center, less than a mile away. He took me inside and I saw that the same nurse was on duty that I had seen earlier that day. She asked me to lie down on a hospital bed and talked privately with the police officer for a few minutes. She asked me for my parents' phone number, and after I had given it to her, she called them and let me talk to them for a few minutes.

The next thing I knew, I was waking up on a mattress in a padded room with wire mesh glass in the windows. It was morning. I did not remember coming to this room. I thought, "They must have drugged me. Where am I? I could be anywhere." I looked out the window but I didn't recognize anything. I suspected I was a prisoner of the CIA, or NSA, or some government agency. I looked out the window again and tried to discern some clue as to where I was. I soon recognized that I was still in a medical facility—but where? Was it the same facility I came into last night?

After a few hours, I got a visitor. It was the same man from the house the night before. He said, "Hi, Kurt. I'm Mr. McKinney, the man whose house you came into last night. Do you remember me?"

I don't remember what we talked about, but his demeanor was calm and concerned. I wondered why he was visiting me. Was he with the CIA? How could that be true? I thought I had gone to his house at random. Maybe I didn't. Maybe they led me in that direction. Maybe they were controlling me with subliminal messages. Maybe everyone in this town worked for the CIA. Maybe this was a secret town. Could that be true?

Soon, a nurse brought me some magazines to read, and I thought perhaps the CIA was trying to communicate with me through the magazines. One had an article about finding a new career. Did they want to hire me to become an agent?

Lockdown

In a little while, another nurse came to the door. I think I had been talking to myself out loud all morning. She said, "Would you like to go out and see where you are? You have to promise me you won't run away. Do you promise not to run away?" I said, "Yes, I promise." She took me down the hallway and outside an exit. She said, "See? You're in Glasgow." I didn't really recognize anything. I thought, "I have to get to my hotel." I started to walk away. She yelled at me, "Where are you going? You said you wouldn't run away! Come back!" I just ignored her. Of course, I wasn't running away, I was *walking* away.

In less than five minutes, a police car pulled up beside me. An officer got out and ordered me into the car. He took me back to the medical center and I was put back into the same padded room.

After perhaps half an hour I started to have another hallucination. The car horns had returned. I started to hear a sound like dozens of cars blowing their horns. It sounded like it was coming from outside the hospital. Soon, it became more intense. It sounded like a thousand cars blowing their horns. It was a very loud sound.

I came to the conclusion that people were blowing their horns for me. They wanted me to be released. I thought, if I don't get out of here soon, there's going to be a riot. I needed to escape. The next time a nurse came to the door, I forced my way past her and ran out of the building. By that time, the sound of the horns had stopped. But when I was outside, I didn't notice that there weren't a thousand cars out there. Once again, the police intercepted me and took me back to the hospital. A short while later, a nurse came to the door and said,

"Tomorrow, your parents will be here. They're coming for you."

Later that day, a mental health worker came to evaluate me. She tried to interview me.

"What is your name?"

"Kurt Snyder"

"Who is president of the United States?"

"Bill Clinton"

"Why are you here?"

"I don't know"

"Where do you think you are?"

"I don't know. I thought I was in Glasgow, Montana, last time I checked . . . but I'm not sure where we are exactly."

"What were you doing last night?"

"I was walking around town."

"Why did they bring you to the medical center?"

"They said they were getting me some help."

"You remember Mr. McKinney? You went into his house last night. Why did you go into his house?"

"I had something in my hand. I had to get it out. I didn't think they were home."

"Are you hearing voices when there is no one there?"

"No."

"Do you think you have any special powers that no one else has?"

"No."

"Do you think you know anything that no one else knows?"

"No."

"Do you want to hurt yourself or other people?"

"No."

"Do you see things that other people don't see?"

"No."

"You ran away from the hospital earlier. You told the nurse you wouldn't run away. Why did you run away?"

"I didn't run away . . . I walked away."

"Why are you here in Glasgow?"

"I came out here on vacation."

As I was being interviewed, I knew what I had experienced, but I didn't have any perspective on why they had brought me to the medical center.

Returning Home

My parents arrived the next day, and a day or two later, I was released under their care on the condition that I be evaluated at a psychiatric institution. My parents took me back to Maryland by plane, and immediately I was admitted to a mental health institution in Baltimore. I stayed there for two or three days. After one day, I was already asking to be released.

A doctor at the institution prescribed anti-psychotic medication for me, but I didn't want to take it. I asked what the medication would do to a normal person, but the doctor couldn't tell me—he said he didn't have any information about that. I certainly wasn't going to take it—who knew what that medication would do to me?

My parents soon came to take me home. They had obtained the prescription the doctor had ordered, but I never took any of the medication. I merely pretended to take it to ease their concern. Even so, my psychotic symptoms decreased somewhat over the next few weeks.

I still thought every day about surveillance, and about the experience I had had in Chicago. I knew something was wrong. I knew that even though I had *thought* people were following me, I didn't actually have any evidence of this. I decided to test myself. I needed to go to a place where everyone I saw was a stranger. I took a morning train up to New York City and walked a few blocks to a park. I made notes about the people I saw on the street. After a little while, I noticed that I thought more than half the people I saw were with Them. Another quarter were "suspicious." This didn't make me question my delusion, but it made me think that I had become conditioned to believe people were with Them.

By June of 2000, I thought it was time for me to go back to work. I had not done any productive work for at least six months. I had quit working as a handyman, so I got a job working for a temporary employment agency in Washington, DC. I soon found that I couldn't work effectively. I wondered constantly if my coworkers, my employers, and random people I met while working were affiliated with Them, the CIA, the FBI, or Congress. My delusions clouded my perception of reality so completely that I couldn't perform any job function that required me to interact with other people. After a short while, I was fired.

At about this time, I started to experience a new dimension of my illness. I became acutely aware of certain stimuli that normal people don't usually notice. Noises like fans running, people coughing, car horns, machinery rattling, tires screeching, wind blowing, engines running, and birds chirping became very disturbing to me. I also became aware of the many movements people make without thinking. People rubbing their chins, scratching themselves, running their fingers through their hair, wiping their noses, and blinking all seemed to gesture very overtly to me in a way they never had before. All these types of stimuli seemed to have some kind of special meaning, as if they were intended to communicate something to me, but I could never figure out what that was.

The Big Picture

Schizophrenia can be a deeply disquieting experience, not only for the individual who has it, but also for others who are touched by the illness. When you have schizophrenia, it's as if your perceptions and thoughts have come loose from their moorings, leaving you adrift in a sea of disorienting and sometimes disturbing stimuli. As a result, you may act in ways that are confusing and even distressing to other people. It may not be until later, after treatment has begun to take hold, that you're able to fully appreciate the effects of your actions on yourself and others.

While you're still out of touch with reality, though, it is nearly impossible to function optimally at home, school, or work. Mentally, you're operating in your own private world. What you see, hear, and touch may be different from what's perceived by those around you, and your interpretations of those perceptions may follow a logic all your own. It's very difficult to understand or adapt to everyone else's reality when you're experiencing something quite different.

That's not to say that people with schizophrenia never have any control at all over their behavior. In fact, most do have some degree of control, and with great effort, some can partially suppress their symptoms for short periods of time. However, the amount of self-control that can be exerted over the illness varies from person to person, and within a particular individual, from day to day. No matter how hard the person tries, sooner or later those suppressed hallucinations and bizarre behaviors are apt to bubble up to the surface unless treatment intervenes.

Travels With Schizophrenia

Having schizophrenia doesn't mean you can't also enjoy traveling once your condition is stable. These pointers can help:

- Talk to your psychiatrist or therapist about your travel plans. Discuss any concerns you may have, and ask whether your medications might need to be adjusted to compensate for the upheaval in your daily schedule. If you're ever advised to postpone a trip for health reasons, listen to that advice.
- Bring enough medication to cover your entire trip as well as a few extra days, in case there is any change in plans. Your health insurance company may allow early refills if you call them and tell them about your upcoming trip.
- Pack your medications in a carry-on bag, since checked baggage can be lost or delayed. To simplify getting through security checkpoints, keep all medications together in a pouch or pocket in your bag, don't fill medication containers too densely, and make sure all medications are clearly identified.
- Travel with someone you trust. Make sure your travel companion is familiar with your treatment plan and knows what to do in an emergency.
- Bring some comforting items from home. Your favorite sweater, an old bathrobe, or pictures of loved ones can make you feel more at ease in unfamiliar surroundings. This helps reduce travel-related stress.

How Does Schizophrenia Affect Everyday Life?

Schizophrenia drives a wedge between the person who has the illness and the rest of society. In fact, for many teenagers and young adults, one early warning sign of schizophrenia is giving up existing relationships with family and friends. Once the illness takes hold, many people with schizophrenia have trouble con-

...one early warning sign of schizophrenia is giving up existing relationships with family and friends.

necting with others on more than a superficial level. Making new friends becomes much more difficult than it once was, and keeping them can be even harder.

Whether at home, school, or work, people with schizophrenia act in accordance with reality as they perceive it. The problems arise when their view of reality doesn't mesh with everyone else's. At times, this may lead to behavior that is restless, almost frantic; they are always on the lookout for the next threat lurking around the corner. At other times, it may lead to behavior that is very withdrawn and detached from the rest of the world. In either case, the actions of someone with schizophrenia may seem strange and inexplicable to other people, who don't understand the skewed perceptions and distorted logic that are driving the behavior.

Other Faces of Schizophrenia

Schizophrenia affects the ability to function at home, school, or work and to relate to other people, but the specific form it takes is as individual as a fingerprint.

- "I was in high school in Canada when my thinking became dark and chaotic. I didn't know what was wrong with me; all I knew was fear. I could not trust anyone, not even my parents, and I thought people were trying to poison my food. Then a strange fog came over my brain. Clarity was absent, and I had concentration issues. I had to limit myself to one class a day in school."—Kevin

- "One day when I was 22, I woke up, and the program on the radio was talking about me. I was really, really scared and confused. My body shook with fright. Then I started really isolating myself. I wouldn't talk to anyone except for professors, the people I volunteered with, and maybe one or two friends I truly trusted. I was living with my dad, and I didn't even talk to him. But I couldn't hide from the voices. After a

(continued)

while, the frequency and duration of the voices increased, and so did the volume. They started following me wherever I went. Even when there wasn't a soul around, I still heard voices. Some were violent, prisoner-type voices telling me, 'You're a man, you're a man.' Others were seductive female voices saying, 'We know what kind of man you are.' And some were saying, 'We're going to get you'—all these paranoid-type things. It was downright harassment."—Leon

- "I started to have psychotic thoughts when I was in college. My particular psychotic thought was that one of my professors was trying to poison me, and by eating some chalk, I could stop the poison from working. Now my boyfriend knew this didn't make any sense, and he knew that there was something wrong, but he continued to stick by me. But the thoughts just didn't let up. I thought people were talking about me when they weren't. I thought everybody was out to get me—that the world was an unfriendly place, and nobody cared about me."—Nikki

- "I was 14 years old when I started having hallucinations. Once at night, I was awake and alone in a room when I saw a raped girl who committed suicide standing near the closed door. She was shouting and crying. It was like a heart attack for me. After several hours, she finally disappeared."—Maya

To others, people with schizophrenia may seem extremely distractible or incapable of paying attention to what's going on around them. In truth, though, the person may sometimes be concentrating quite intently on private thoughts and perceptions. Imagine a classroom filled with students. A few are doubtless thinking about the lecture, while others are concentrating on the cute student sitting next to them or daydreaming about their plans for the evening. But a student with schizophrenia may be totally preoccupied with trying to decipher the coded messages that they believe the teacher is sending by blinking her eyes.

Needless to say, this type of disconnect between internal thought and external reality can have wide-ranging consequences. At home, teenagers or young adults with schizophrenia may grow distant from parents and siblings, let chores and homework slide, or start neglecting their personal appearance. At school or work, their performance may drop off dramatically. Even once–star performers may begin failing classes or getting fired from jobs.

While it's ideal if help is sought in the early stages of the illness, that doesn't always happen. And even if a professional is consulted, the correct diagnosis may not be immediately apparent. Instead, the earliest symptoms are often blamed on more common conditions, such as depression, anxiety, or drug or alcohol abuse. By the time a full-blown psychotic break occurs,

...the earliest symptoms are often blamed on more common conditions, such as depression, anxiety, or drug or alcohol abuse.

however, the problems are greatly magnified. The person's behavior is apt to be quite disruptive, and on occasion, it may be destructive to property or dangerous to that individual or others. At this point, inpatient care in a psychiatric hospital is usually needed.

When and Why Is Hospitalization Helpful?

When you're feeling healthy and doing well, a hospital may not sound like a very appealing place to be. Yet when you're acutely ill with a serious disease, it's often the best and safest place to receive intensive treatment and recover as quickly as possible. Schizophrenia is no exception. In fact, more than half of those who receive inpatient psychiatric care each year are diagnosed with schizophrenia. Decisions about hospitalization are made on a case-by-case basis. Typically, though, hospitalization may be recommended for schizophrenia if you:

- Pose a threat to yourself or others
- Are unable to care for yourself
- Are behaving in a very bizarre or destructive manner
- Require medication that must be closely monitored for a while
- Need round-the-clock care to get severe symptoms under control

Inpatient care may be provided in the psychiatric unit of a general hospital or in a specialized psychiatric hospital operated by a private company or government agency. When you're admitted to a hospital, an extensive evaluation is done. This allows the professionals there to develop a treatment plan that's specially geared to your individual needs. The goal is to help you regain your mental equilibrium and resume your life outside the hospital as soon as possible.

Inpatient treatment usually involves a combination of medication and psychotherapy, both one-on-one with a therapist and in a group with other patients. Group meetings can be especially encouraging, because it's often a tremendous relief to discover that other people have been going through similar experiences. (More information about these treatment options can be found in Chapter 4.) Many hospitals also provide related services. For instance, occupational therapy helps patients learn the skills they'll need for daily living outside the hospital. Recreational therapy uses activities such as arts and crafts, games, dance, movement, and music to improve overall well-being and help patients hone their social skills.

...it's often a tremendous relief to discover that other people have been going through similar experiences.

There are several advantages to receiving treatment in a hospital. Since some people try to hurt themselves or others because of their illness, one major benefit is 24-hour monitoring to keep patients safe until their condition is more stable. At the same time, it's easier to do in-depth medical and psychological testing in a hospital setting. If a new medication is prescribed, trained staff can adjust the dose until it's just right, as well as watch for side effects. If alcohol or drug abuse is also a concern, this problem can be addressed along with the mental illness.

If You're Feeling Suicidal

When your logic is twisted by schizophrenia, hurting yourself can sometimes seem to make sense. In addition, depression often goes hand in hand with schizophrenia, whether as a result of the brain disease itself or as a consequence of accepting that you have a serious illness. The tragic result is that suicide is the number one cause of premature death in people diagnosed with schizophrenia. Sadly, an estimated 6% to 15% of people with schizophrenia die by suicide.

Just because suicide is common among people with schizophrenia doesn't mean it's okay to hurt yourself, or that experiencing suicidal thoughts is unavoidable. If you ever find yourself thinking seriously about suicide or feeling the urge to hurt yourself, take action right away:

- *Tell someone you trust.* It's best to choose an older person—such as a parent, doctor, school counselor, school nurse, or clergyperson—who has more experience to draw upon when handling this type of situation.
- *Seek professional help.* Suicidal thoughts are an urgent symptom that needs immediate attention. If you're already in treatment, call your psychiatrist or therapist. If not, ask a trusted adult to help you find mental health care.
- *Call for help and hope.* Another source of immediate, 24-hour assistance is the National Suicide Prevention Lifeline (800-273-TALK).

On the downside, a hospital is the most expensive place to receive treatment, so even if you're lucky enough to have insurance, convincing the insurance company to pay for inpatient care isn't always easy. Hospitalization also involves the greatest curtailment of your freedom to do as you please. But keep in mind that the average length of stay for adults in a psychiatric hospital is just 12 days. When you're suffering from severe symptoms, the benefits of intensive treatment in a hospital usually far outweigh the temporary limitations on your activities.

...keep in mind that the average length of stay for adults in a psychiatric hospital is just 12 days.

What Are the Ins and Outs of Inpatient Care?

A large majority of adults in psychiatric hospitals are there voluntarily. Adults can also be admitted involuntarily, but only under very specific circumstances. Even then, legal safeguards are in place to protect civil liberties. Most states allow a physician to order involuntary hospitalization for a short evaluation period, usually three days. After that, if the evaluation team believes a longer hospital stay is needed, it can request this at a court hearing. In the hearing, the state must show that certain criteria have been met. One situation in which adults can be involuntarily hospitalized is when they pose a danger to themselves or others. In some states, involuntary hospitalization also is permitted for adults who are so gravely disabled that they're unable to make rational treatment decisions for themselves.

If you're under 18, the situation is a bit more complicated. Some states have extended adult-like legal protections to adolescents younger than 18. But elsewhere, parents may be able to sign a minor into a psychiatric hospital without the minor's consent if the admission is deemed appropriate. A neutral fact-finder still must review and approve the admission. Rather than a judge or hearing officer, though, this fact-finder may be a mental health professional.

Regardless of your legal status, if you're ever in a situation where psychiatric hospitalization is recommended, it's wise to take that advice to heart. Schizophrenia itself can distort your judgment and sap your motivation to seek help. It also may make it harder to trust other people, such as your parents or psychiatrist, who are making treatment decisions on your behalf. As difficult as it might be to accept, however, hospitalization is often needed to get severe symptoms under enough control that you can begin working on your recovery.

INSURANCE ISSUES

Sometimes the biggest obstacle to getting hospital care is financial rather than legal. If you and your family can afford to pay for an expensive inpatient stay out of your own pockets, this may not be an issue. Most families aren't so fortunate, however. If you have health insurance, it's smart for you or your parents to ask about the mental health benefits *before* a crisis occurs. Keep in mind that many insurance plans provide less coverage for mental health services than for other medical or surgical services. For example, many cover an unlimited number of days in the hospital for medical or surgical care, but cover only 30 to 60 days a year for mental health care. Some insurance plans also require higher copayments and deductibles for mental health care, and other plans set lower annual and lifetime spending limits.

If you don't have insurance through your parents or an employer, you might qualify for services through Medicaid or the State Child Health Insurance Program (SCHIP). Medicaid is a joint federal-state government program that provides health insurance to eligible low-income and disabled individuals. SCHIP is another federal-state program that provides coverage for uninsured children and teenagers (ages 18 and younger) in lower-income families who aren't eligible for Medicaid. Compared to private insurance plans, these government programs tend to provide relatively generous coverage for mental health services. However, you and your family must meet eligibility criteria to qualify. To find out more about the programs in your state, start with GovBenefits.gov (800-333-4636, www.govbenefits.gov) and Insure Kids Now! (877-543-7669; www.insurekidsnow.gov).

Whether you have private or public insurance, chances are good the insurance company uses some form of managed care, a system designed to keep the cost of health care down. One common managed care strategy is utilization review, which is a formal review of health care services to determine whether payment for them should be authorized or denied. To make this determination, the managed care company considers two factors: whether the services are covered under the insurance plan and whether they are medically appropriate and necessary. In other words, the managed care company must be convinced that the ill person's condition is serious enough to require inpatient care before it will authorize payment. Even if the admission is approved, it's usually just for a limited stay. The patient's progress is then reviewed periodically to determine whether the stay should be extended.

Inpatient care is costly. As a result, managed care companies are sometimes reluctant to approve hospitalization or to extend the stay for as long as might be optimal. But if care is denied, the psychiatrist and the patient or patient's parent can appeal the decision. To find out more about the appeals process, contact the member relations department at your managed care company. It often pays to be persistent when it comes to getting hospitalization covered.

It often pays to be persistent when it comes to getting hospitalization covered.

Where Can You Get Help Outside the Hospital?

From the day you enter the hospital, the staff will start planning for the day you leave. Outside the hospital, it's vital to keep up your treatment. Depending on your needs and what's available in your community, this treatment can be provided in several settings:

- Residential treatment center—A treatment facility where you live in a dorm-like setting with a small group of people. The treatment there is less specialized and intensive than in a hospital, but the stay may last considerably longer.
- Partial hospitalization—A treatment option where you spend at least four hours a day on therapy and other treatment-related services, but go home at night. A wide range of services may be provided, such as individual or group therapy, special education, job training, and therapeutic recreation.
- Outpatient treatment—A treatment option where you live in the community as usual, but occasionally see a doctor or therapist.

Most of the treatment that people with schizophrenia receive actually occurs outside a hospital. In the next two chapters, you'll learn more about the various treatments and support services that are available. The better use you make of outpatient services, the less likely it is that you'll need to be an inpatient in the future.

These paintings are by people who have or may have had schizophrenia.

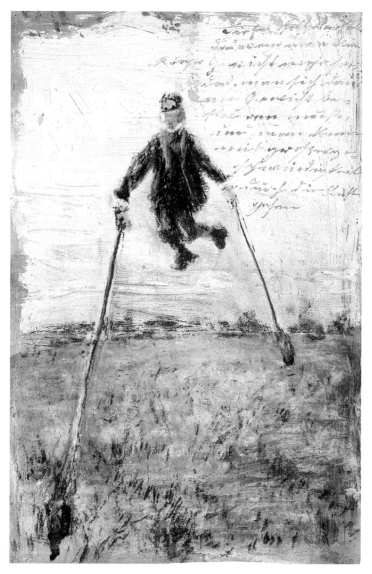

Man on Stilts, by German artist Josef Forster (composed after 1916). The Prinzhorn Collection, Heidelberg, Germany

Untitled drawing of a man by Portuguese artist Jaime Fernandes (1899–1968). Collection ABCD, Paris

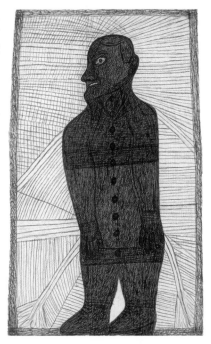

World Axis with Hare, by German artist August Natterer (1868–1933). The Prinzhorn Collection, Heidelberg, Germany

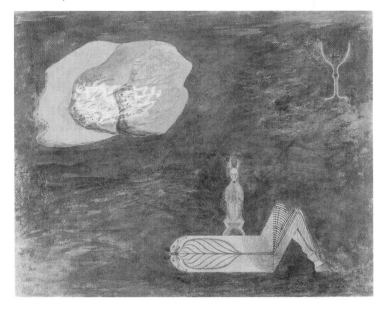

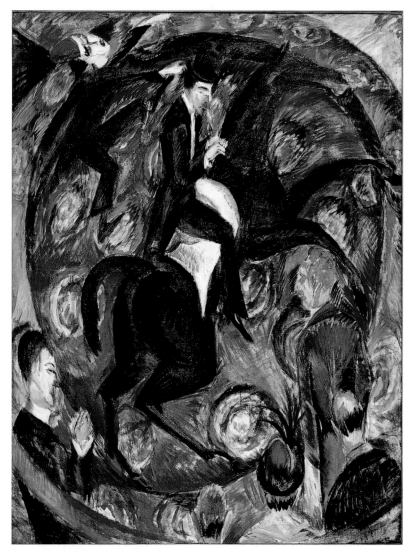

Circus Rider, by German artist Ernst Ludwig Kirchner (1880–1938).
Saint Louis Art Museum, Bequest of Morton D. May

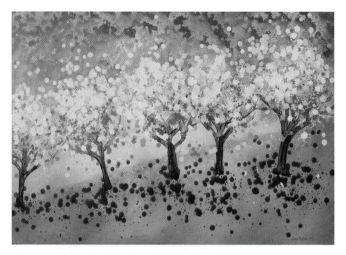

Five Trees, by contemporary American artist Jerome Lawrence. Collection of Jerome Lawrence

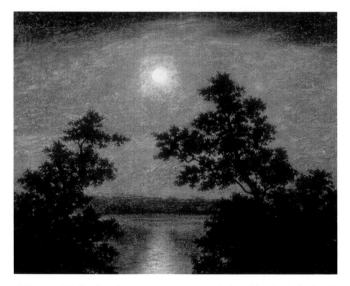

Silvery Night, by American artist Ralph Alfred Blakelock (1847–1919). Gift of Marion Sharp Robinson, from the permanent collection of the Utah Museum of Fine Arts

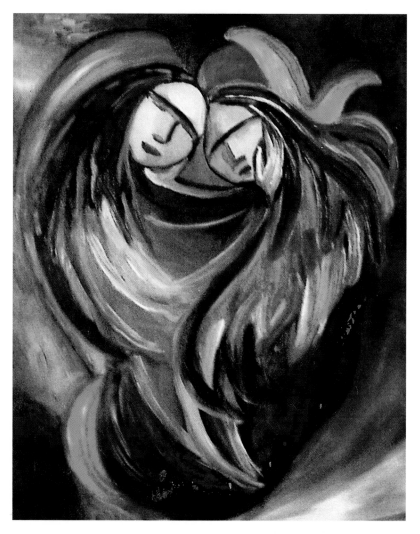

Two Angels, by contemporary American artist Suzanne Schneider.
National Alliance for Research on Schizophrenia and Depression
Artworks

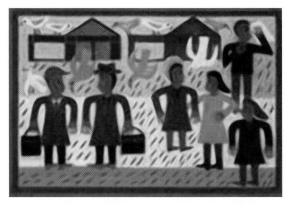

Six Figures with Pigeons and Buildings, by American artist Eddie Arning (1898–1993). Smithsonian American Art Museum/ Art Resource, New York

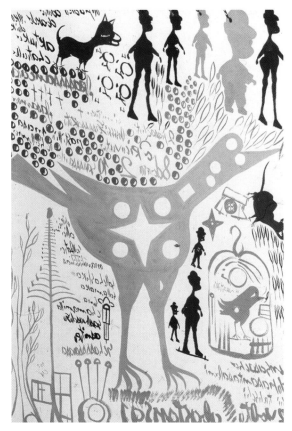

Untitled painting by Italian artist Carlo Zinelli (1916–1974). Judy A. Saslow Gallery, Chicago

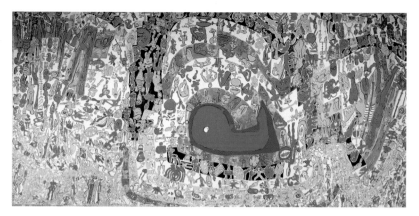

Embryonic Madness, by contemporary American artist Linda Carmella Sibio. Courtesy Andrew Edlin Gallery, New York

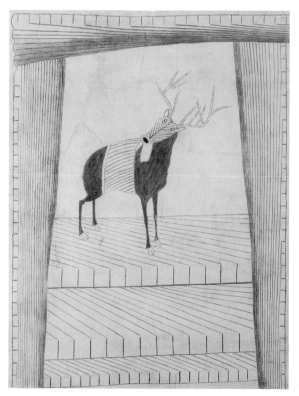

Untitled drawing by Mexican artist Martin Ramirez (1895–1963). Collection ABCD, Paris

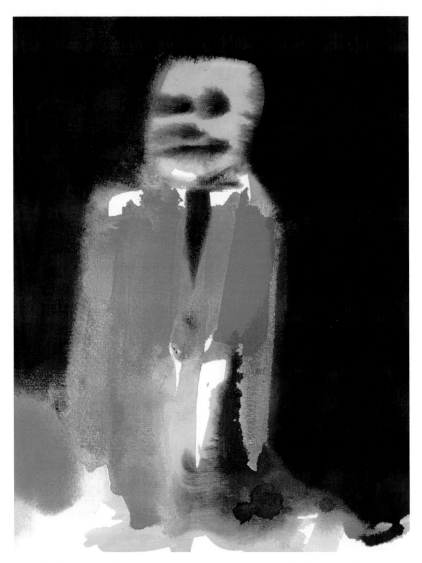

Untitled painting by contemporary American artist Harold Plople.
National Alliance for Research on Schizophrenia and Depression
Artworks

Chapter Four

Naming and Facing the Enemy: Diagnosis and Treatment

My Story

Chronologically, the periods between my severe psychotic episodes were becoming shorter. My first episode happened in August of 1999. The next one was in March of 2000, seven months later. Now, it was only three months past March, and I was starting to become psychotic again. I was entering a phase where my normal delusions were supplanted by new ones that seemed to emerge from nowhere. My imagination almost completely replaced reality with its own storyline about the universe.

I was driving home one day when my mind became disorganized. I couldn't decide what to do. I was consistently making wrong turns on my way to my house. I started to believe the CIA was somehow controlling my thoughts with subliminal and inaudible messages piped into my truck with a hidden speaker. I thought they were trying to dictate my route home. I decided that I would drive a semi-random route home, instead of letting them control me. I would only make a turn in the direction of my house if the last digit of the minutes on the digital clock read 1, 3, 5, or 7. Otherwise, I would continue straight ahead. As you can probably guess, it took me a *very* long time to get home.

After arriving at the house, I started reading a book I had purchased several years earlier. I wondered if the book had been published only for me, and whether the music CDs I often listened to were produced just for my benefit. I call this phenomenon "personalization." I have often read that sometimes people with schizophrenia believe that random things have personal significance just for them.

The Delusions Intensify

Later that day, at dinner time, my mother introduced me to some exotic pears. They were very different from the common pears I was accustomed to eating. I thought to myself, "Maybe they are the result of genetic engineering." I didn't think this kind of thing was possible yet. Immediately after this, I thought, "Maybe I'm 25 years in the future!" Schizophrenic delusions tend to have permanence even when they don't make sense. I thought, "My parents look the same. How could I be in the future?" It occurred to me that the people I saw in front of me might be clones of my parents. How could I tell if they were my real parents? Even I look the same myself. How could I still look the same after 25 years? Maybe somehow my body was preserved for all those years. I pondered this for at least a half an hour, but finally decided I wasn't really in the future. But it took an awful lot of thought to convince myself it wasn't true.

That night, I became fearful that the CIA was going to break into the house and kill my parents. I would be blamed for it. I stayed awake the entire night.

> Schizophrenic delusions tend to have permanence even when they don't make sense.

Very early that morning, I had an unusual experience. I was thinking deeply about my own thoughts and how one thought leads to the next. I started to see a glowing multi-colored light in the corner of the room, but there weren't any lights turned on. This was another hallucination, but I didn't know it at the time. My thoughts seemed to merge together, as if looping back on themselves, but then they seemed to stop completely. This was accompanied by a strange sound, like a drop of water falling into a pool, except the sound was very loud. It was like nothing I have ever experienced before or since, and the sensation was very strange. I'm trying to relate it to you now because sometimes people with schizophrenia may have unusual mental experiences that defy description, that may seem very unlikely when they try to communicate the experience to the average person. I wondered at this point whether I might have brain damage. These peculiar mental experiences may be interpreted by people with schizophrenia in strange ways. They may believe someone or something else is controlling their thoughts, or inserting thoughts into their head.

Back to the Hospital

My parents were aware that I was having another severe psychotic episode, so they arranged to have me admitted to the hospital again. On the way there, we stopped at a fast-food restaurant. There was a man in the restaurant moving very slowly. My attention was focused on this one man. Why was he moving so slowly? "My god!" I thought. "I've somehow caused time to slow down! What have I done to cause time to slow down?" We left the restaurant and everything seemed normal, but this idea stuck in my brain. I thought, "We must be caught in some space-time bubble where time is moving normally, but the rest of the world must be in this horrible predicament where time is moving slowly!" We arrived at the hospital about 40 minutes later, and they put me in an isolation room and locked the door.

While I was in isolation, I began to think about what (I thought) I had caused. I thought that people might think I was God because I had caused time to slow down. I believed that some, being Christians, might want to crucify me to see if I would come back to life. I became very anxious and nervous. I had to escape! I tried to break through the wall of the room, but the staff came in and strapped me to a table. In a short while, they transferred me to a locked psychiatric ward.

Back to the Outside World

After a few days, I was released. I still felt that I needed to work. This time, I got a job at a coffee shop in Annapolis, a few minutes away from my house. I lasted one week before they fired me. To this day, I don't exactly know why.

Smoking cigarettes was an escape for me. I had started smoking a few years earlier. My girlfriend at that time smoked occasionally, usually when we were at a bar, and I picked up the same habit. At first, it was just one or two cigarettes a month. But as my mental health deteriorated, I started smoking much more often. When I was psychotic, I would sometimes smoke four or five cigarettes in a row while I was trying to sort out what was real from what wasn't.

While I was sucking on a cigarette, I would forget about the turmoil in my mind. The effect never lasted longer than the cigarette, but it was a few minutes of calm, or at least a reduced state of anxiety. I was putting my future health in jeopardy, but those cigarettes tasted so damn good.

Back then, I thought I could control how much I smoked and when. The frequency with which I smoked increased so gradually that I never noticed I was becoming addicted. If I could go back in time, that's something I definitely would change. Had I never tried that first cigarette, I would never have developed a craving for one. As I've since discovered through three failed quit attempts, it's a lot easier to never start smoking than it is to stop.

As I've since discovered through three failed quit attempts, it's a lot easier to never start smoking than it is to stop.

Giving **Them** *a Name*

I had been assigned to a new psychiatrist, who diagnosed me for the first time with schizophrenia. Now, five years later, I find it amazing that he correctly diagnosed me. I never told him anything about my feelings or my thoughts. He made the diagnosis based on the testimony of my family.

Schizophrenia—the word just bounced off me. Schizophrenia was a mental disorder. I certainly didn't have schizophrenia. I didn't have a mental disorder. How could the doctor know what was happening to me? He wasn't in the CIA or FBI. He never worked at the facility. He couldn't know the truth about me. Right? I forgot what I was told as soon as I left the doctor's office.

A few weeks later, I had a second appointment with the same psychiatrist. I was not taking the medication he prescribed. I think he knew this. He demanded that I take the drug— Geodon. He said he could not be my doctor if I didn't take it. I eventually decided to follow his recommendation, but my decision was based in part on a delusion that They would stop following me if They thought I was crazy—if I took the medicine, I would seem to be crazy, and They would have no need to follow me anymore. The surveillance would stop. Ironically, it was the truth.

The Big Picture

How Is Schizophrenia Diagnosed?

The key to diagnosing schizophrenia is a mental status exam. This exam often is performed by a psychiatrist, a medical doctor who specializes in the diagnosis and treatment of mental illnesses and emotional problems. The psychiatrist asks questions designed for two purposes: to find out what problems a person is having and to consider other possible explanations besides schizophrenia. Because a person who is currently psychotic may have trouble communicating, family members and friends might be asked to fill in missing information.

The questions typically cover:

- Personal background, such as family, friends, living situation, school or work, and hobbies
- Current symptoms, including how they've changed over time and how long they've lasted
- Previous mental or physical disorders
- Any family history of mental illness

In addition to asking questions, the psychiatrist looks for other clues about how the person is doing. For example, is the person clean and dressed appropriately for the weather? Is the person alert and focused? What do the person's tone of voice, facial expressions, and body language convey?

One question that's usually asked is, "What drugs are you taking?" Street drugs such as LSD and PCP can produce hallucinations, delusions, and disordered thinking, and marijuana sometimes leads to paranoid thinking and strange bodily sensations. In addition, a number of prescription medicines occasionally cause hallucinations or delusions as a side effect. This question can help sort out psychotic symptoms caused by schizophrenia from those produced by drugs, so it's important to answer honestly.

A complete diagnostic workup also includes a medical exam to look for other diseases that can cause symptoms similar to those of schizophrenia. Examples of such diseases include brain tumors, viral encephalitis, epilepsy, multiple sclerosis, and AIDS. Depending on which alternate diagnoses are being considered, the doctor might order lab tests to analyze samples of blood, urine, or cerebrospinal fluid, the fluid surrounding the brain and spinal cord. In addition, the doctor might sometimes order magnetic resonance imaging (MRI), a powerful imaging technique that uses magnets and radio waves to produce pictures of the brain, or an electroencephalogram (EEG), a diagnostic technique that produces a graphic record of the brain's electrical activity.

A psychological evaluation might be done as well. Typically, it's performed by a psychologist, another type of mental health professional who provides assessment and treatment for mental and emotional disorders. Psychological tests assess intelligence, personality, or specific mental abilities, such as concentration, memory, and judgment. Depending on the particular test, it might involve answering questions out loud or on paper, drawing a certain shape, repeating a string of words, or solving puzzles.

What Conditions Often Coexist
With Schizophrenia?

Of course, diagnosis isn't always an either/or proposition. Some people with schizophrenia have one or more other disorders at the same time. When this happens, diagnosis and treatment can get a little more complicated. Still, for the best results, it's important that these other conditions be diagnosed and treated, too. Below are some of the conditions that often exist side by side with schizophrenia:

- Substance abuse—The abuse of drugs and alcohol is considerably more common in people with schizophrenia than in the population at large. In fact, studies have found that 40% to 70% of people with schizophrenia also have a history of substance abuse or addiction. Among the most commonly abused substances are alcohol, marijuana, and cocaine. Nicotine addiction is an issue for many as well. It's estimated that about 80% of people with schizophrenia are smokers, and those who smoke tend to do so heavily, averaging 30 cigarettes a day.

    The reason for such high rates of substance abuse isn't clear. But it's thought that some people with schizophrenia may abuse drugs or alcohol in an effort to soothe their symptoms. There's just one flaw in this plan: It doesn't work. In the long run, substance abuse can actually increase symptoms and interfere with treatment. Plus, when people with

In the long run, substance abuse can actually increase symptoms and interfere with treatment.

schizophrenia abuse drugs or alcohol, they increase their risk of suicide, homelessness, jail, and physical health problems.

Coffee and a Cigarette

Many people with schizophrenia always seem to have a cigarette or cup of coffee in their hand. Both the nicotine in cigarettes and the caffeine in coffee are powerful drugs. They're known to affect the levels of various brain chemicals, which, in turn, might influence some symptoms. In the case of cigarettes, there are also nicotine receptors in the brain that may play an important role.

As with other drugs, one theory is that people with schizophrenia may smoke or drink coffee in an attempt to self-medicate. There's evidence that this strategy might indeed help people temporarily feel better in some ways. For example, one study of 50 smokers, half with schizophrenia and half without, found that smoking enhanced attention and working memory in those with schizophrenia but not in the other smokers. Other research has suggested that smoking may normalize the way certain genes work in people with schizophrenia.

By the same token, both nicotine and caffeine can affect the action of antipsychotic medications. Smoking *lowers* blood levels of most antipsychotics. This effect is especially pronounced with clozapine and olanzapine, which could reduce how well they work. In contrast, caffeine substantially *raises* blood levels of these two drugs, which could increase unwanted side effects.

Both smoking and excessive coffee carry their own health risks as well. Smoking is a major cause of cancer, heart disease, stroke, and lung disease, and it also has been linked to everything from cataracts and peptic ulcers to sexual problems in males and infertility in females. Drinking coffee to excess can produce not only "the jitters," but also insomnia, muscle twitching, rapid heartbeat, upset stomach, and rambling thoughts and speech.

The bottom line: There are much healthier, more effective ways of coping with schizophrenia, so smoking and drinking large amounts of coffee definitely aren't recommended. But if you do have a cigarette or coffee habit, be sure to tell your doctor. That way, your medication dosage can be adjusted accordingly.

- Depression—About 75% of people with schizophrenia have at least one episode of major depression. This is more than just feeling blue or down in the dumps now and then. Major depression is a serious disorder that involves being in a low mood nearly all the time, or losing interest or enjoyment in almost everything. People with depression typically feel sad, empty, and hopeless, but teenagers sometimes feel irritable instead. These feelings last for at least two weeks and cause significant distress or problems in everyday life. They're also associated with other mental and physical symptoms, such as a change in eating or sleeping habits, lack of energy, feelings of worthlessness, trouble with concentration, and thoughts of suicide.

> People with depression typically feel sad, empty, and hopeless, but teenagers sometimes feel irritable instead.

- Anxiety disorders—People with schizophrenia have a higher-than-average risk of anxiety. These disorders are characterized by excessive fear or worry that is long-lasting or recurrent and interferes with everyday life. In particular, schizophrenia has been linked to higher rates of panic attacks and obsessive-compulsive disorder (OCD). Panic attacks are sudden, unexpected waves of intense fear and apprehension that are accompanied by physical symptoms, such as a racing or pounding heart, shortness of breath, and sweating. OCD is characterized by repeated, uncontrollable thoughts that cause anxiety as well as repetitive actions that the person feels driven to perform in response to these thoughts.

Why Is Professional Treatment So Important?

Contrary to what you may have heard, schizophrenia is a highly treatable disease. Unfortunately, many people with schizophrenia find it hard at first to accept the help they need. They may not believe anything is wrong, because their delusions or hallucinations seem quite real to them. Or they may be reluctant to take medication for a long time, especially if unwelcome side effects occur. Yet when people finally begin taking their medication as prescribed and working hard at therapy, the improvement can be dramatic. While there's no cure for schizophrenia yet, there *are* effective ways of managing symptoms and easing the return to everyday life.

The first step toward getting better is finding the right professional help. Several different types of professionals provide mental health care. In addition to psychiatrists and psychologists, there are clinical social workers, psychiatric nurses, and mental health counselors. Often, a psychiatrist oversees the medication side of treatment, while another mental health professional provides therapy.

Treatment has two goals: reducing symptoms right now and preventing psychotic episodes in the future. In general, the earlier treatment begins, the more effective it's likely to be. Medication is essential for getting severe symptoms under control. Once the symptoms have lessened, a combination of medication and therapy can be very helpful. Getting appropriate treatment can make the difference between losing touch with the world and living successfully in it.

A Brief History of Schizophrenia Treatment

In the first half of the twentieth century, people with schizophrenia often lived out their days in mental institutions. By the 1940s, however, the media had begun to publicize the deplorable conditions in some of these places. *Life* magazine published an exposé titled "Bedlam 1946: Most U.S. Mental Hospitals Are a Shame and a Disgrace," and *Reader's Digest* published a condensed version of *The Snake Pit*, a novel that recounted the disturbing experiences of one hospitalized woman.

Then in the 1950s, chlorpromazine and reserpine, the first effective medications for treating schizophrenia, were introduced. During the next decade, activists began calling for reforms in society's treatment of mentally ill individuals. Thanks to the new medications, it was time to rethink the future for many who in earlier days would have been consigned to an institution for life.

The stage was set for a movement called deinstitutionalization, which involved the widespread release of individuals from mental institutions. The goals of this movement were valid and humane. In fact, most people with schizophrenia and other mental illnesses *can* live in the community with proper treatment and support. Unfortunately, the sudden outpouring of people from mental hospitals overwhelmed the system. Without adequate care and assistance, many mentally ill individuals fell victim to homelessness, poverty, and crime.

In the short term, deinstitutionalization was disastrous for many. Today, community resources have still only partially caught up to the demand, and there continues to be room for improvement in access to care and support services. Yet the coming decades are poised to bring great treatment advances that you and future generations can take advantage of.

What Medications Are Used to Treat Schizophrenia?

Antipsychotic medications are used to treat the symptoms of schizophrenia. They can be quite effective at decreasing positive symptoms, such as delusions, hallucinations, bizarre behavior, and disorganized thoughts. In general, they're less effective when it comes to negative symptoms, such as apathy, withdrawal, and lack of emotion. Because each person with schizophrenia is different, though, no single medication works well for everyone. If you're prescribed an antipsychotic, it might take a few tries to find the best one at the most appropriate dose for you.

There are two basic categories of antipsychotics. First-generation, or "typical," antipsychotics have been around since the 1950s, while second-generation, or "atypical," antipsychotics were introduced in 1990. Scientists still don't know exactly how these medications work. However, all affect the dopamine system within the brain. Specifically, these drugs fit into certain dopamine receptors, keeping dopamine from attaching there and having its effects.

OLDER ANTIPSYCHOTICS

First-generation antipsychotics are thought to work by adjusting dopamine levels in the brain. Examples include Haldol (haloperidol), Navane (thiothixene), Prolixin (fluphenazine), Stelazine (trifluoperazine), Thorazine (chlorpromazine), and Trilafon (perphenazine). Although these older medications tend to be as effective as newer ones, they're more likely to cause unpleasant side effects, such as muscle stiffness, abnormal movements, tremors, and restlessness. Yet they work well for some people and typically cost less than newer medications.

NEWER ANTIPSYCHOTICS

Second-generation antipsychotics have fewer side effects than their first-generation cousins, so they're often the treatment of choice today. These newer medications block not only certain dopamine receptors, but also serotonin receptors. The significance of the latter effect is still being debated, though. Some scientists believe that serotonin does indeed play a key role in schizophrenia. But others believe that what really sets apart the newer antipsychotics is not their effect on serotonin at all, but the speed with which they detach from dopamine receptors once they've done their job there. Research is currently underway to sort out this issue.

The first of the newer antipsychotics was Clozaril (clozapine). It's especially helpful for people with severe schizophrenia who haven't responded to other treatments. However, it also has the potential to cause agranulocytosis, a disorder in which bone marrow doesn't produce enough white blood cells to fight infection. To monitor this risk, people taking Clozaril must have a blood test every week or two. Obviously, that's a big drawback. But for those who aren't helped by other medications, the benefits may be well worth the extra cost and inconvenience.

Several other second-generation antipsychotics have since been introduced. Each has its own unique set of side effects (see the table on the next page). Most of these side effects are mild, and many lessen or disappear within a few weeks. Some people with schizophrenia felt the side effects of older medicines were as bad as the disease. These newer antipsychotics have changed the lives of innumerable people by offering the possibility of effective treatment without such distressing side effects.

OTHER MEDICATIONS

Antipsychotics are the mainstay of schizophrenia treatment. However, other types of medication are occasionally used as

Second-Generation Antipsychotics

Trade Name	Generic Name	Most Common Side Effects
Abilify	aripiprazole	headache, weakness, nausea, vomiting, constipation, anxiety, problems sleeping, lightheadedness, sleepiness, restlessness, rash
Clozaril	clozapine	drowsiness, increased salivation, rapid heartbeat, dizziness, constipation, headache, shaking, lightheadedness
Geodon	ziprasidone	feeling unusually tired or sleepy, nausea or upset stomach, constipation, dizziness, restlessness, diarrhea, rash, increased cough or runny nose
Risperdal	risperidone	anxiety, uncontrolled movements, constipation, nausea, upset stomach, runny nose, rash, vision changes, saliva increase, abdominal pain, inability to control urination, weight gain
Seroquel	quetiapine	headache, agitation, dry mouth, constipation, pain, vomiting, upset stomach, weight gain
Zyprexa	olanzapine	sleepiness, dry mouth, dizziness, restlessness, constipation, upset stomach, weight gain, increased appetite, tremors

Less Common but Serious Side Effects

- Neuroleptic malignant syndrome—A life-threatening nervous system problem that can affect your kidneys. Symptoms include a high fever, stiff muscles, sweating, fast or irregular heartbeat, change in blood pressure, and confusion. Get medical help right away if you develop these symptoms.
- Tardive dyskinesia—A disorder causing repeated, involuntary, purposeless movements that can develop after many months or years of taking antipsychotic medications. Examples of the movements include grimacing, smacking your lips, sticking out your tongue, blinking your eyes, or moving your fingers. This problem is more common with first-generation antipsychotics. Call your doctor right away if you develop muscle movements that you can't stop.
- High blood sugar and diabetes—If you have diabetes, your blood sugar should be checked frequently.

well. For instance, people with schizoaffective disorder may need a mood stabilizer—a drug that helps even out severe mood swings—in addition to their antipsychotic medication. In other situations, an antipsychotic might be combined with an anti-anxiety medication to help manage anxiety or agitation, or with an antidepressant to help relieve depression.

TIPS ON TAKING YOUR MEDICINE

- Be realistic about what you expect. People differ in how quickly they see results. Some symptoms might improve within days, but others might take weeks or months to get better. As a rule, though, you can expect to see considerable improvement by the sixth week. If you don't, your doctor might adjust your treatment plan.

...you can expect to see considerable improvement by the sixth week.

- Use memory aids to help you remember your medication. Mark off each dose on a calendar, or use a weekly pillbox with separate compartments for each day so you can see at a glance if you've taken your pills. If forgetting your pills is still a problem, ask your doctor whether you might be able to take your medicine in the form of a special injection that has an effect lasting up to a month, known as depot medication. While convenient, not all antipsychotics are available in this form.

- To avoid harmful drug interactions, tell your doctor about any other drugs you're taking. This includes not only other prescription medications, but also nonprescription medicines, vitamins, herbal supplements, alcohol, and illegal drugs.

- Talk to your doctor about troublesome side effects. Your doctor may be able to change your dosage, adjust when you take it, switch you to a different medication, or prescribe an additional treatment to keep the side effects under control.

- Let your doctor know right away if your symptoms start to return. Symptoms may flare up again from time to time, no matter how careful you are about following your treatment plan. No one will blame you for a recurrence. However, it's important to deal with the symptoms as soon as possible, before they get out of hand.

- Never stop your medication without consulting your doctor. Even if you're feeling perfectly fine, it may be necessary to stay on medication to keep feeling that way.

Other Faces of Schizophrenia: "Mark"

Mark has been on medication since 1994, when he was diagnosed with schizoaffective disorder at age 18. He's doing well now, but finding the right medication for him took some trial and error. "I started with Haldol in the hospital," he says. "It knocked me out—totally took away all my energy. All I wanted to do was sleep, but when you're in the hospital, they try to force you to stay awake during the day hours, so it was very, very difficult." Mark then switched to a different drug, which wasn't much better than the first. Finally, he switched to a third, which was much more effective, and had minimal side effects. In addition to the antipsychotic, Mark is currently on a mood stabilizer to even out his mood swings.

(continued)

At first, Mark resisted the idea of taking medication long-term. "I would go off my medication as soon as I felt well, but then I would get really sick and wind up in the hospital again. After a while, I just said to myself, 'Okay, here are the facts: If I don't take my medicine, I'm going to end up back in a place where I don't want to be. If I do take my medicine, I won't end up there anymore.'" On Mark's current medication, the side effects are milder, but they haven't disappeared completely. Mark still struggles with some tiredness and weight gain. Yet he now believes the pluses of sticking to his treatment plan far outweigh these minuses.

Mark also believes in the benefits of speaking up. "If you don't feel like your medication is working for you, it's perfectly fine to talk to your doctor about it," he says. "My advice is to have an open dialogue with your doctor—and never forget what would happen if you didn't take anything."

How Does Psychological and Behavioral Therapy Help?

Once someone with schizophrenia is in stable condition on medication, adding psychological and behavioral therapy to the mix can help that person learn valuable skills for handling the disease. For example, let's say a person is having trouble with communication, relationships, and motivation. By learning new skills for coping with those areas, it's more likely that the person will be able to attend school or hold a job, as well as enjoy a satisfying social life.

...a good therapist can provide information, understanding, and encouragement—three key ingredients for recovery.

In addition, research has shown that people with schizophrenia who receive regular psychological and behavioral therapy in addition to drug therapy are more likely to stick to their medication schedule. They also tend to have fewer relapses and hospitalizations than those who don't receive such help. That's not surprising, since a good therapist can provide information, understanding, and encouragement—three key ingredients for recovery. Below are brief rundowns of the types of therapy that are most commonly used for schizophrenia.

SUPPORTIVE PSYCHOTHERAPY

Supportive psychotherapy refers to "talk therapy" in which the goal is to strengthen people's coping skills and provide them with reassurance. It's different from the type of therapy that aims to probe deeply into psychological conflicts, which has not proved to be useful for treating schizophrenia. Supportive psychotherapy, on the other hand, has proven to be exactly what its name implies: a helpful source of emotional and practical support for many schizophrenia patients.

In supportive psychotherapy, discussions focus on problems and decisions that a person is facing here and now, rather than on conflicts rooted in the past. The therapist can help identify realistic solutions to problems, offer encouragement as progress is made, and sustain the person in times of crisis. Talk therapy is no substitute for medication. But when a supportive relationship with a therapist is combined with drug therapy, it may provide added benefits.

BEHAVIOR THERAPY

Behavior therapy focuses on changing or replacing unwanted behaviors. This form of therapy uses the principles of learning theory to strengthen adaptive behaviors while helping people unlearn maladaptive ones. Let's say a person is having trouble making conversation. Rewards, such as praise or special privileges, might be used to teach basic conversational skills one at a time; for example, maintaining eye contact, standing at an appropriate distance, speaking at an appropriate rate, and using facial expressions that match what's being said. Once these basic skills have been mastered, the person might move on to more complex ones; for example, starting a conversation, asking questions, giving information, and expressing feelings through words. Step by step, the person develops helpful new behavior patterns.

COGNITIVE THERAPY

Behavior therapy is often paired with cognitive therapy, which focuses on correcting inaccurate patterns of thinking. Cognitive therapists can help people with schizophrenia learn how to test the accuracy of their beliefs. Other possible goals of cognitive therapy include learning how to tune out auditory hallucinations and using self-talk to help shake off apathy and depression. When paired with medication, cognitive and behavior therapy seem to be effective at decreasing symptoms.

GROUP THERAPY

Sometimes therapy takes place one-on-one between a therapist and a patient. At other times, though, a group of people with similar problems will work on specific issues together under the guidance of a therapist. This is known as group therapy. Many teenagers and young adults feel more comfortable talking in a group of people their own age, and group therapy may be ideal for them. However, others are more at ease with one-on-one therapy, and that's fine, too.

FAMILY THERAPY

In family therapy, several members of a family participate in therapy sessions together. Living with schizophrenia can be quite stressful not only for the person who has it, but also for that person's family members. Therapy might help some families find better ways of interacting with each other, keeping stress under control, and helping one another cope with the disease, day in and day out.

As you can see, psychological and behavioral therapy for schizophrenia tend to be down-to-earth and focused on developing practical skills. Often therapy may be provided in conjunction with a rehabilitation program. Such programs help people regain any life skills they've lost; for example, the skills needed to socialize, cook,

...psychological and behavioral therapy for schizophrenia tend to be down-to-earth and focused on developing practical skills.

clean, budget, shop, hold a job, and solve everyday problems. Rehabilitation programs also help people learn useful new skills; for example, the skills needed to manage their illness and the stress that goes along with it. You can find more information about this type of psychosocial rehabilitation program in Chapter 5.

While psychological and behavioral therapy may be helpful, you can't just talk yourself out of having schizophrenia any more than you can talk yourself out of having diabetes or asthma. Schizophrenia is a biologically based brain disease, and as such, it calls for a biologically based treatment—in other words, medication. Yet behavioral and psychological treatments also have their place. When added to medication, they can give people valuable life skills as well as the hope and motivation that are required to put those skills to the best possible use.

TIPS ON MAKING THE MOST OF THERAPY

- Expect to be an active participant. Therapy isn't something that's done for you. It's something you do

for yourself under the guidance of a trained professional. The more you put into it, the more you'll get
back out.

- Give therapy a chance to work. Like schizophrenia
itself, therapy is an ongoing process. Unfortunately,
there aren't any quick fixes for schizophrenia, so
progress may occur in small steps instead of giant ones.
- Talk to your therapist if you ever start feeling dis-
couraged. It's important to let your therapist know
if you have any concerns about how therapy is going. That way, you'll be able to work on the problem
together.

One last word of advice: The professionals on your treatment
team can only help if you show up for appointments. It's
tempting to skip appointments once you start doing better, but
continued treatment is critical for keeping your recovery on
track and preventing relapses. Schedule your appointments
with treatment providers well in advance, so you'll be able to
plan around them. Then mark all appointments on a calendar as soon as you make them. If you still have trouble remembering, ask a family member or friend to write down
the appointment, too, so they can remind you. Also, line up
transportation ahead of time, if necessary. Keeping appointments may take a little effort, but you'll get a lot of benefit in
return.

What Is the Outlook for the Future?

When you have a chronic medical condition such as diabetes
or high blood pressure, keeping up your treatment over the
long haul is vital for decreasing symptoms and reducing

complications. The same principle holds true for schizophrenia. Current treatments only control symptoms of the disease. They don't cure the underlying problem. Therefore, to maintain progress, most people with schizophrenia probably need to continue treatment for the rest of their lives.

Staying on medication is critical. No one likes the idea of taking medicine indefinitely, but the alternative is much worse. Most people with schizophrenia who go off their medicine have a relapse—in other words, a return of their symptoms—within a year. On the other hand, studies have shown that long-term use of medication can help prevent relapse and promote lasting recovery.

Different researchers define recovery in different ways, so it isn't easy comparing statistics on long-term outcomes from one study to another. Nevertheless, several studies have found that about half of people with schizophrenia eventually recover or substantially improve over a period of two decades or more. Of course, all of the people in those studies were diagnosed at least 20 years earlier. It's quite possible that those being diagnosed today, who have the benefit of the latest treatment advances, will have even higher recovery rates 20 years from now.

The earlier treatment is started, the better the chance of recovery seems to be. Antipsychotic medications are most effective during the first psychotic episode, when they significantly improve symptoms in three-quarters of people who take

Antipsychotic medications are most effective during the first psychotic episode ...

them. As time goes on and psychotic episodes mount, treatment becomes less effective. That's why it is so important to seek help without delay.

Even if you start treatment early and continue it faithfully, you may never be exactly the same as you were before schizophrenia. However, it's important to keep that fact in perspective. Schizophrenia doesn't have to be an end. By combining medication with psychological and behavioral treatment, you can learn to adapt and move on.

Chapter Five

Beating the Enemy: Recovery From Schizophrenia

My Story

I started taking antipsychotic medication regularly in July 2000. Almost immediately, it seemed to prevent the most severe symptoms of psychosis. But at first, it did nothing to control my long-standing delusions—which by this time I had had for several years.

Also, after about a month of taking the medication, I started to experience a very unusual side effect. I could not walk with a normal gait. I could only shuffle along, using baby steps, like an old man might do. I reported this to my psychiatrist, and he made an adjustment to my medication. This side effect eventually disappeared.

After a few more months on the medication, I developed a deep depression. This was the lowest point of my life. I had lost all interest in the world around me, all my mental and physical energy. My motivation to achieve anything at all was gone. I stayed in bed for most of every day for more than one month.

It was autumn. At one point, I went outside to try to rake leaves, but I couldn't. Every task seemed to require a huge amount of energy that I didn't have. After a few minutes, I gave up trying and went back inside to my bed. I felt great despair, sadness, and fear. How could I spend the rest of my life this way? I had no hope for the future. It seemed to me that I would feel this way forever. I thought I would never achieve anything significant ever again.

I knew at this point that I was experiencing mental illness, as far as my depression was concerned. I knew that my behavior and mental status weren't normal. Other people weren't lying in bed all day like I was doing. However, I still did not believe that I had been insane, and I *certainly* didn't believe that I had schizophrenia. Depression was an acceptable diagnosis for me, but schizophrenia was not.

Depression was an acceptable diagnosis for me, but schizophrenia was not.

During my depression, I couldn't imagine anything that would make me feel better. Nothing seemed to give me pleasure. Life soon became dreary, dark, and miserable. I slept as often as possible in an attempt to escape the dread of existence. At least when I was asleep I didn't have to face reality.

After consultation with my psychiatrist, he prescribed an antidepressant for me. Within six weeks, my depression was gone.

About this time, I also started to experience a new symptom of schizophrenia—inappropriate affect. This is when you have an abnormal emotional response to a certain stimulus. For example, after my grandmother died, I had the urge to laugh when I was telling people about her death even though I was actually very saddened by it. I certainly didn't think it was funny and I didn't want to laugh about it. But in my brain, somehow, the outward response of laughter was connected with the wrong feeling inside me—sadness. It was a problem that

I tried hard to suppress, and I felt guilty about this tendency for several weeks. Eventually, the problem went away and has not returned since.

Accepting Schizophrenia

I had been taking antipsychotic medication for several months when I slowly came to terms with the fact that I had a serious mental illness. I started to question some of my beliefs and thought processes. At first, only the most bizarre delusions seemed implausible. Certainly I had never caused time to slow down. My life wasn't fabricated by a virtual reality machine run by aliens. I couldn't have been transported into the future. However, my longer-held delusions were more resistant to reason. It took me over a year to admit to myself that I wasn't being followed by people working at the facility, or the CIA, or the FBI. Those delusions just seemed more plausible to me. They evaporated only after I had convinced myself that I did in fact have a severe mental illness.

The first time I really accepted that I had schizophrenia was when I finally realized that some of my experiences had been hallucinations. I remembered the sound of a thousand cars blowing their horns, and I remembered that when I went outside, there were not a thousand cars out there. I remembered seeing the glowing light in the corner of the room when there were no lights turned on. Remembering these experiences helped me to accept that I had symptoms of schizophrenia (hallucinations), and this knowledge made me question whether I had other symptoms of the disease (delusions). I finally understood the inaccuracy of my belief that people were following me in Chicago. I came to understand that the town of Glasgow had not been evacuated. I was never a candidate for a secret job at the CIA or FBI.

The most important thing I did to get myself healthy was to take the medication. I don't think I would have ever realized that I was experiencing abnormal thought patterns if I hadn't.

When I realized that I had a mental illness, I was very ashamed of myself for several months. I had always thought I was a smart person. How could I become mentally ill? The truth is, there is no correlation between intelligence and mental illness. Anyone can be afflicted by mental illness, regardless of their intelligence. Eventually, my shame disappeared when I realized that I could not have done anything differently in my life. I was not capable of recognizing on my own that something was seriously wrong with me, and therefore I couldn't prevent it from happening. Most of my friends and family who knew about my mental problems were still very close to me—they never abandoned me. This was truly a blessing.

> When I realized that I had a mental illness, I was very ashamed of myself for several months.

A New Direction

Sometime in 2001, I decided that I needed to do something with my life—I needed direction. A friend of mine was working as a database administrator and he suggested that I pursue this career. I had already demonstrated some success in this field by programming the database application for Dan, and the database administrator job seemed like a natural extension of this work. I did some research and learned that I could obtain a certificate as a database administrator if I took a series of five classes and five exams. However, there were two problems—the classes were extremely expensive, and my computer had died the previous month. I had no money to spend because I had not been working for more than six months.

While talking with Dan one day, he told me that he would buy me a new computer, and pay for the first classes I took. I thought, what a generous gift! I accepted it with much appreciation. A short time later, I had passed the first class and the first exam. After this success, my parents decided to help me pay for the remaining classes.

I found the database classes to be very intense and difficult. I could not absorb all the knowledge that was presented to me within the time allotted for the class. I developed a pattern where I would take a class, and then study for the corresponding exam for the next two months. Even then, I did not pass all the exams the first time. I had to take two exams twice. Eventually though, I passed all the exams and was certified as a database administrator. From start to end, the whole process took me about 16 months—probably much longer than required by the average person, but the important thing is that I finished successfully.

That same year, I realized that I needed to do something with my free time that would contribute to the community, so I joined my local volunteer fire department. Originally, my intention was to be an emergency responder. I took a full-time training course for a month to earn the certification to ride the fire engine. The course was very difficult and demanding for me, but I completed it successfully. After responding to a few emergencies, though, I decided that I wasn't good at making decisions in a high-pressure environment. I wondered what to do all the time, and I had a lot of anxiety about emergency situations, so I decided to volunteer as an administrative member instead. The fire department had many opportunities for volunteers besides emergency response, and most of the volunteers did not want to do these other jobs anyway. I became a handyman for the department, doing minor building repairs whenever they were needed. The following year, I was appointed as a trustee to the board of directors, and I was asked to be chairperson of the budget and finance committee. My administrative duties have been increasing every year since, and I find that I can do these types of things very well.

In 2002, I started looking for a job as a database administrator. My mental state had been stable for more than a year, and I was ready to go back to work. A friend of Dan's mentioned that his wife might have a job for me where she worked. I called her office and arranged an interview. I was hired shortly thereafter.

This job was nearly ideal for me. It was a government job, with good benefits, and close to home. In a short while, I had learned nearly everything I needed to know to perform well.

After I had been working in my new job for about a year, I began to experience an unpleasant new side effect of the antipsychotic medication. I started to feel an unusual type of anxiety that was different from anything I had felt before. It was intense and extremely discomforting. I could not concentrate on any task for more than a few seconds, and my job performance was suffering. I had confided in my boss that I had schizophrenia, and she let me go home early on occasion. Unfortunately, the anxiety became so commonplace that I was having it for several hours every day. I certainly couldn't leave work early every day. I reported this to my doctor and he explained that I was probably having akisthesia—an effect of the antipsychotic drugs. This akisthesia is by far the worst emotional feeling I have ever experienced in my entire life. While I was suffering from it, I wanted to escape from existence. If it ever became a permanent feeling, suicide might have seemed like a good option. I can't stress enough how horrible this feeling was. My doctor decided to prescribe a different antipsychotic medication in the hope that this anxiety would diminish, and thankfully it did. We gradually reduced my old medication, and increased the new one. The anxiety was gone within a month.

One side effect that I have been unable to reverse is weight gain. The medication I currently take is known to cause an increase in body weight. So far, I have gained about 30 pounds, an increase of about 15% of my normal mass. However, the advantages of the medication far outweigh this disadvantage. I have no intention of changing it.

The Big Picture

Improvement is a positive thing, of course. Yet the first steps toward improvement from schizophrenia can be jarring. As medication takes effect and your mind begins to clear, it's a shock to realize just how sick you have been. Accepting your diagnosis may take some time.

Once you've accepted your illness, you can fight back more effectively.

One thing that holds some people back is the mistaken belief that acceptance means surrender. In truth, it can mean just the opposite. Once you've accepted your illness, you can fight back more effectively.

Ultimately, the goal is not only to survive, but also to thrive. Years ago, this might not have been a realistic goal for most people with schizophrenia, but today it's within the reach of many. While improved medications are part of the reason, great strides also have been made in nonmedication treatments and supports. Getting this kind of help often makes the difference between merely living with schizophrenia and living well.

What Are Psychosocial Rehabilitation Programs?

Medication is crucial for getting many symptoms of schizophrenia under control and keeping them that way, but it often takes more than just medicine to reclaim a full life and return to the world of school or work. That's where psychosocial rehabilitation programs come in. Such programs provide psychological, social, and job training, which helps people with schizophrenia regain any life skills lost due to their illness as well as develop new skills for managing their disease.

Psychosocial rehabilitation is at the heart of a relatively recent shift in the way professionals look at schizophrenia. The old view held that the best possible outcome was to stop hallucinations and delusions and prevent hospitalizations. The new view holds that such improvements are only the start. Just like anyone else, teenagers and young adults with schizophrenia need to finish school, begin careers, establish grown-up relationships, and learn to live in the adult world. Rehabilitation programs aim to teach the skills that are needed to reach these goals.

Research has shown that people who take part in psychosocial rehabilitation programs while continuing their other treatment tend to manage their illness better than those who don't. Interestingly, studies also have suggested that people with mental illness may think about recovery a bit differently than the professionals do. Rather than focusing on completely getting rid of all symptoms, people with schizophrenia often say they're more interested in being able to live on their own and have a full and rewarding life. They want to accept themselves, be accepted by others, manage any symptoms that don't go away, and take charge of their own well-being. When recovery is defined in these terms, it's clear why psychosocial rehabilitation is so important.

Medication tends to work better for treating positive symptoms of schizophrenia, such as delusions and hallucinations, than for treating negative symptoms, such as not showing emotion, speaking in a monotone, seeming uninterested in the world and other people, and having trouble getting anything done. While delusions and hallucinations may be more dramatic, people with schizophrenia often say it's the negative symptoms that cause the most problems, because such symptoms make it nearly impossible to have the full life they want. Psychosocial rehabilitation plays a critical role here, by giving people the skills they need to cut down or work around their negative symptoms.

What Types of Training and Support Are Available?

The types of services available to people with schizophrenia vary from place to place. In addition, different individuals need different types of training and support. These are some of the training programs and support services that you might find provided along with medication and talk therapy:

- *Case management* is designed to coordinate all the different treatments and services a particular individual receives. It helps the different care providers work together efficiently, and it also helps ensure that all of the person's needs are met. Among other things, case managers may help people line up treatment, financial assistance, and supported work and living arrangements.
- *Social skills training* helps people with schizophrenia develop the skills they need to communicate effectively and interact well with others. Basic skills that everyone needs to master include being an attentive listener,

making requests in a tactful way, and expressing both positive and negative feelings. Other topics that might be covered include making conversation, being assertive, managing conflicts with other people, living with roommates, making friends, going on dates, and interviewing for jobs. Numerous studies have shown that such training can help people with schizophrenia get along better in a wide variety of situations.

- *Independent living skills training* helps people develop the skills they need to live on their own and get along in the world. Examples of such skills include cooking, cleaning, shopping, managing money, applying for a job, dealing with coworkers, using public transportation, and socializing. Also included are the skills needed to solve everyday problems and cope with stress.

- *Supported employment* is a service that helps people with schizophrenia find and keep jobs that pay at least minimum wage in the community and are suited to their interests and abilities. Because schizophrenia usually strikes during the prime years for finishing school and starting a career, it can seriously limit a person's ability to find a meaningful job. Yet most people with schizophrenia say they want to work, and this type of program helps them overcome any barriers standing in their way. Employment specialists guide the person with schizophrenia through finding a job, succeeding in the workplace, and handling any challenges that arise.

- *Illness management training* is geared toward helping people with schizophrenia develop personal strategies for coping with their disease. Typically, it consists of weekly sessions that last about three to six months. The sessions may be provided individually or in a group. In these sessions, people learn practical facts about mental illness that help them make more informed decisions about their own care. They also learn how to use their medication properly and manage their symptoms more effectively. In addition, they're taught how to recognize the early warning signs of a relapse so they can respond quickly, before the symptoms get too out of hand.

- *Family psychoeducation* helps people with schizophrenia team up with their family members so they can work together toward recovery. Although the term *family* is used, close friends may participate as well. Typically, five or six people with schizophrenia and their families meet regularly over a period of at least six months to learn about the illness and develop coping strategies. For the person with schizophrenia, this type of program has been shown to promote recovery, lead to higher rates of employment, and reduce the need for hospitalization. For the family as a whole, it can reduce stress and help mend strained relationships.

- *Peer support centers* are places where people with mental illness can drop in to socialize. They're safe spots to hang out, watch TV, play games, get to know other people with similar concerns, and stay off the street. In addition, they're good places to find informal support and help. Some centers also offer organized activities and field trips or host self-help groups and training classes.

- *Self-help groups* bring together people with schizophrenia so they can share support, encouragement, and hands-on advice. A good starting place for finding self-help groups in your area is the online directory of the National Mental Health Consumers' Self-Help Clearinghouse (www.cdsdirectory.org). Schizophrenics Anonymous is one particular self-help organization that now has more than 160 groups meeting in 31 states (www.nsfoundation.org/sa, 800-482-9534).

Your treatment provider can point you toward resources in your area, or you can call your local chapter of the National Alliance on Mental Illness (NAMI; www.nami.org, 800-950-6264) or the National Mental Health Association (NMHA: www.nmha.org, 800-969-6642) to ask about what's available.

ASSERTIVE COMMUNITY TREATMENT

For people with very severe and long-lasting symptoms, one of the most effective approaches is assertive community treatment (ACT). In ACT, a team of professionals works together to provide comprehensive treatment and support that are tailored to the individual needs of a person with schizophrenia. ACT is intended to help those who are having the most trouble taking care of themselves, staying safe, finding a decent place to live, and holding a job. These individuals have needs that aren't adequately met by less intensive services, and without extra help, many have problems with unemployment, substance abuse, and homelessness.

A typical treatment team is composed of 10 to 12 professionals, such as psychiatrists, nurses, psychotherapists, social workers, employment specialists, and substance abuse counselors. The approach differs from case management in a key respect. Case managers arrange for services that actually are provided by other agencies or clinics. The professionals on the ACT team provide the services themselves, so they're able to offer more personalized care. They also keep the schedule flexible. When a problem comes up, the person with schizophrenia can get help right away without having to wait for an appointment.

In ACT, there is no predetermined set of services or arbitrary time limit on how long a person can stay in treatment. The team tries to provide whatever it takes to help the person with schizophrenia live in the community and work toward getting better. Services are available 24/7, and in the beginning, some people are in contact with their team members several times a day.

Numerous studies have compared ACT to ordinary case management. These studies have shown that people who receive ACT are less likely to be hospitalized and more likely to have a stable place to live. Research also has found that people who receive ACT and their families tend to prefer it to a more traditional approach. While ACT isn't for everyone, it can be invaluable for those whose symptoms don't respond to less intensive styles of treatment.

How Can You Cope With Schizophrenia at School?

Because schizophrenia affects the workings of the brain, it often has a major impact on the ability to get along at school. The exact effects vary depending on the type and severity of symptoms a particular student has. Among other things, schizophrenia may create problems with concentrating, interacting with others, handling negative feedback, adjusting to change, and filtering out distractions.

If you're struggling at school as a result of having schizophrenia, there are steps you and your parents can take to get your education back on track. The most important step is getting proper treatment for your illness, including taking any medication as prescribed. Beyond that, though, you may find

...you may find that certain changes in the classroom can go a long way toward helping you do your best.

that certain changes in the classroom can go a long way toward helping you do your best. Remember: The goal isn't to lower the standards for your education or get you out of doing hard assignments. Rather, the goal is simply to help you work up to your potential.

FOR HIGH SCHOOL STUDENTS

When all you need are relatively minor classroom changes, an informal meeting between you, your parent, and your teachers may be all it takes to set things in motion. You or your parent should be prepared to share information about what schizophrenia is (and isn't), which symptoms you're currently having, and how they're affecting you at school. To request more extensive changes—for instance, placement in a special class or specialized skills training—you'll probably need to go through a more formal process. Up through high school, two federal laws may come into play when you request special educational services based on having a disability:

- Individuals with Disabilities Education Improvement Act of 2004 (IDEA)—To qualify for services under IDEA, you must show that you have a disability that impacts your ability to benefit from general educational services. This requires going through an evaluation and being labeled as having an "emotional disturbance." The process is lengthy and involved, but it can be well worth the effort if you have extensive and long-lasting needs. If you qualify, you'll receive an individualized education program (IEP)—a written educational plan

Sample Adjustments at School

Sometimes relatively small changes can make a big difference in your ability to succeed at school. The exact changes you might need will depend on the symptoms you have. Below are examples of the kinds of adjustments that some students with schizophrenia have found very helpful.

Common Problem	Possible Solution
For all students	
Having trouble tuning out distracting sights and sounds	Moving to a seat farther away from the source of distraction
Feeling anxious over being in a classroom with the door shut	Being allowed to sit close to the door or an open window
Having a dry mouth as a side effect of medication	Being allowed to keep a bottle of water at your desk
Feeling very restless and unable to sit still during lectures	Getting advance permission to take short breaks when necessary
Becoming extremely stressed out when taking tests	Being allowed extra time or taking the test in a less stressful format
Losing focus or becoming fatigued when taking a lengthy exam	Dividing the exam into segments that can be spread out over a few days
Having trouble composing your thoughts in a formal essay	Being given the option to substitute a recorded presentation
Getting confused easily when given oral instructions for completing assignments	Receiving advance, written notice of assignments so you can plan ahead
Having trouble writing by hand as a side effect of medication	Typing papers or test responses on a computer instead
Feeling sluggish or having trouble focusing in the morning	Starting later in the day or scheduling the most important classes in the afternoon
For college students	
Having trouble registering or applying for financial aid	Receiving help with these complicated but necessary procedures
Feeling disoriented and ill at ease on an unfamiliar campus	Receiving a tour that helps you get your bearings, plan how to get to class, and know where to turn for help
Being unable to carry the usual course load for full-time status	Being classified as full-time despite taking a reduced number of courses
Becoming tired or overwhelmed by the logistics of getting to class	Being provided with a parking pass or elevator key
Failing to finish all required coursework by the end of a semester due to a relapse	Receiving an "incomplete," which usually means you don't have to pay again or retake the course to complete it

that spells out how your individual academic needs will be met. For more details, visit the Web sites of the U.S. Department of Education (idea.ed.gov) or the Parent Advocacy Coalition for Educational Rights (www .pacer.org).

- Section 504 of the Rehabilitation Act of 1973—To qualify for services under Section 504, you must have a physical or mental impairment that substantially limits one or more major life activities, such as learning, thinking, communication, and self-care. Clearly, most students with schizophrenia meet this standard. The 504 process is faster and more flexible than the one required under IDEA. In addition, there is sometimes less stigma attached to having a 504 plan than an IEP. On the other hand, schools don't get extra funding under Section 504 the way they do under IDEA, so this route may not be appropriate if you need costly services.

FOR COLLEGE STUDENTS

Section 504 applies to college students, too, as does Title II of the Americans with Disabilities Act of 1990. Both of these laws prohibit discrimination on the basis of a disability. However, you should be aware of some important changes in your educational rights once you graduate from high school.

Section 504 requires school districts to provide a "free appropriate public education" to each young person in their jurisdiction up through high school age. After high school, this requirement no longer holds. Nevertheless, colleges can't deny you admission simply because of a disability, assuming you otherwise meet their standards to get in. Colleges also must provide appropriate academic adjustments to ensure that they don't discriminate on the basis of a disability.

Examples of possible adjustments include reducing a student's course load, substituting one course for another, or allowing extra time for tests. However, there are limits to the types of adjustments that colleges are required to make. For instance, they don't have to make courses easier, provide personal tutoring, or make changes that lead to undue cost or administrative work.

It's always your decision whether or not to notify your college that you have schizophrenia. Of course, you'll need to take this step if you want to request an academic adjustment based on your illness. Then you'll need to go through the school's request procedure, and you will probably be required to submit documentation showing that you have a disability affecting your academic performance. All of this can take time. Therefore, even though you can request an academic adjustment at any time, it makes sense to start the process as early as possible.

> It's always your decision whether or not to notify your college that you have schizophrenia.

Almost every college has a person on staff—often called the Section 504 coordinator, ADA coordinator, or disability services coordinator—who can answer your questions about disability issues. For more information, you can also contact the U.S. Department of Education's Office for Civil Rights (800-421-3481, www.ed.gov/ocr).

How Can You Deal With Schizophrenia at Work?

Once you're ready to enter the workforce, you're likely to face a whole new set of opportunities and challenges. The ADA is the main federal law governing disability issues at work. This law gives civil rights protections to individuals with disabilities that are similar to those provided to individuals on the basis of race, color, sex, national origin, age, and religion. When it comes to the workplace, Title I of the ADA states that businesses must make "reasonable accommodations" to protect the rights of people with disabilities in every aspect of employment, from the application process and hiring to wages, benefits, and promotion.

Just as with students, employees are considered to have a disability if they have an impairment that substantially limits at least one major life activity. The ADA also applies to employees who have a record of such impairment, such as those who have recovered from a mental illness. Like anyone else, employees with disabilities must have the necessary skills, experience, and training to do what they were hired to do. The law simply says that employers must make reasonable accommodations—adjustments to a job or the work environment that enable a qualified person with a disability to perform the essential functions of his or her job.

Employers are not allowed to ask about a disability during the hiring process. They can only ask about your *ability* to do the work. After you're hired, employers aren't required to make accommodations until they know about your disability. If you think an accommodation would help you do a better job, consider speaking up. Any accommodation will have to be individualized to your particular needs and situation. Organizations such as the U.S. Department of Labor's Job Accommodation Network (800-526-7234, www.jan .wvu.edu) often can suggest low-cost solutions to common problems.

Keep in mind that there are limitations to what employers are required to do. For instance, they aren't required to make changes that would impose an undue hardship on the business. Also, the ADA only applies to businesses with 15 or more

Joining a Clubhouse

One way of easing into employment is by joining a clubhouse, which is a place where people with mental illness can slowly adjust to a work-centered day. Under the guidance of staff, members do all the work that's needed to run the clubhouse, such as clerical work, data input, and meal preparation. Eventually, members move into short-term, entry-level jobs in the community. The idea is to gain some experience, learn how to get along at work, and try out different types of jobs. The ultimate goal is to move on to more permanent jobs, but studies that have looked at whether members achieve this goal have found mixed results. Still, some people do seem to benefit from taking a gradual approach to entering the world of work. If you're interested in learning more, the International Center for Clubhouse Development has a directory of clubhouse programs on its website (www. iccd.org).

employees. Further information is available from the U.S. Department of Justice (800-514-0301, www.ada.gov).

What Are Options for Living on Your Own?

Growing up, you probably looked forward to the day when you could move out of your parents' house and into a place of your own. Having schizophrenia doesn't necessarily mean you can't realize your dream, but it does make the task of living on your own a little more complicated. Now when you're choosing a place to live, you need to consider not only how much it costs and how far it is from your school or job, but also how much assistance you'll need and how close you'll be to treatment providers and support services.

One possibility is to continue living a while longer with your parents or another family member. This works out well for some families, who can serve as a ready-made support system while you focus on progressing at school or work and moving

Sample Accommodations at Work

You can find solutions to many work problems with a little effort and creativity. Job accommodations need to be individualized, based on both your symptoms and the nature of your job. These are examples of the kinds of accommodations that some workers with schizophrenia have found very helpful.

Common Challenge	Possible Solution
Keeping your energy up throughout the whole day	Longer or more frequent work breaks
	Flexible hours or a part-time schedule
	Work schedule starting later in the day to counter morning fatigue
Concentrating on the details of your job	Periodic rest breaks to refocus
	Partitions around your work space to reduce distractions
Doing a series of tasks in the proper order	Written instructions for the tasks
	Checklists to help you keep track of where you are in the sequence
	Additional training time, if needed
Finishing projects and meeting deadlines	Daily to-do list for checking off tasks as you complete them
	Prominently displayed calendar with deadlines marked
Working well with your supervisor	Open communication about problems
	Written short-term and long-term goals
	Regular meetings to discuss progress
Adjusting to a new work environment	Advance notice about upcoming changes
	Gradual introduction of a few changes at a time
Handling stressful situations at work	Work breaks to de-stress as needed
	Permission to call treatment providers and other supporters during work hours, if necessary

toward recovery. For other families, though, it leads to considerable stress. In that sense, it's no different from the experience of young adults without schizophrenia. Some have a relaxed relationship with their parents, and others have more conflict, even when there is lots of love underneath.

If you're a young adult, and you and your treatment provider think it's time for you to strike out on your own, there are several housing options available. They offer a range of supervision and help, depending on how much assistance you need at any given time. At first, you might need considerable support until you learn the ropes of caring for yourself. As you develop skills and confidence, you may gradually move toward more independent living.

For those needing the most support, there are living facilities with trained professionals on hand 24 hours a day. A step below that are group homes and boarding houses where a group of people with mental illness live together with a supervisor who doesn't have formal training in mental health care, but who can help out with practical matters. The next step down are houses and apartments where a case manager or other mental health professional stops by periodically to see how things are going. For some people, this winds up being a good long-term arrangement. Others move on to living completely independently, either by themselves or with roommates, without the need for formal supervision.

There are also government housing programs available to help with the rent when necessary. The specifics vary from state to state. However, in so-called Section 8 programs, the tenant pays some portion of his or her income toward the rent and receives a voucher to make up the difference. In Chapter 9 programs, the landlord receives a subsidy in exchange for providing housing to people with disabilities. Your caseworker or the housing coordinator at your rehabilitation program can help you find the best housing option for you.

Other Faces of Schizophrenia: "Nikki"

By the time Nikki graduated from college, it was apparent that something was seriously wrong. She was having paranoid delusions and behaving erratically. "My mom kicked me out of the house," she recalls. "My boyfriend tried to help by moving me into his parents' house. I lived there for about five years—this was from 21 to 26 years old. During that time, I had a dozen or so jobs, but at each job, I was let go. Sometimes it was a matter of hours, and sometimes it wasn't until months later, but I couldn't hold onto a job for anything."

Nikki continues, "My boyfriend started to get really depressed, because he didn't know what to do. He went to a counselor for himself, and as he was describing our life, the counselor said, 'It sounds like your girlfriend might have schizophrenia.'" That was a big awakening for him. He got on the Internet and found out about schizophrenia, and he realized that the symptoms matched what he was seeing in me. He was seeing a lot of apathy and weird behavior. So he got me to a doctor, and the doctor said I had schizoaffective disorder."

Nikki was referred to an intensive, five-day-a-week therapy and rehabilitation program. "Before that, one symptom of my illness was that I couldn't make eye contact with people. Also, because I thought people were saying bad things about me, I would avoid talking to them." She credits the program with helping improve her social skills. She also learned about managing other symptoms, such as lack of motivation and hearing voices. "Four times a day, we would meet in a group for about an hour to talk about different subjects—like one subject was Schizophrenia Focus, where we would talk about the symptoms of schizophrenia and what to expect. I had experienced all these symptoms without knowing what they were, but once I started learning more about them, everything started to gel for me."

Despite the new insights, Nikki found that there weren't any shortcuts to recovery. "Therapy was like rolling a large rock up a hill inch by inch every single day," says Nikki. "I learned that you have to celebrate your baby steps, because that was the only way to get through it. For me, it was a very slow process—it took five years—but I did eventually get better."

After the first couple of years, Nikki began to yearn for a more independent lifestyle. "It dawned on me that I didn't know how to cook, I didn't know how to clean. I used to know how to do those things when I left my mother's house for college, but the illness just took everything from me." Determined to relearn those skills, Nikki moved into a nonprofit group home. "Every day, I did two chores, one in the morning and another in the afternoon," says Nikki. For example, she would take out the trash, wash the dishes, cook a meal, or clean and mop the bathroom, kitchen, or foyer.

After two-and-a-half years in the group home, Nikki was ready to move into an apartment of her own. That was three years ago. Today she works as a substitute teacher and teacher's aide. These are on-call positions, so if she's going through a stressful period and her symptoms are flaring up, she'll turn down jobs until her symptoms are under better control. Nikki also is active as a mental health advocate, speaking to high school and college audiences about her recovery from mental illness.

To minimize flare-ups, Nikki keeps close tabs on her lifestyle. "I keep a journal of how much I eat, how much I exercise, and how much I sleep each day," she says. "I also write on a calendar what I did some days, like if I had an appointment or went to see somebody. When my symptoms flare up, sometimes if I look back at my calendar, I can see that I was stressed out over a situation, and that gives me some insight into why I was feeling the way I did at a particular time. Then I try to prevent the same thing from happening again by doing something differently in the future."

Nikki still sees her longtime boyfriend on the weekends. "We try to go places that are relaxing, like the seashore, which is only about a 45-minute drive away," she says. "I've long recognized that the bar scene is not for me, because I can't drink alcohol with my medication and it's kind of stressful, so my boyfriend knows not to take me to places like that."

"Before I got sick, I was planning to go to medical school," Nikki says. "Mental illness did change a lot of things in my life, and I had to give up that goal. But all in all, I think it has made my life a lot richer. I've had to live more deliberately and in a more holistic way. I'm no longer caught up in the details of things. I'm more mature in my outlook on life."

What Are Tips for Handling Social Situations?

Schizophrenia can be a lonely experience. During psychotic periods, a person may literally be living in a separate reality. Even after the delusions and hallucinations pass, negative symptoms—such as trouble showing interest in other people or difficulty expressing emotion—can make social interaction difficult. It may take a conscious effort to rebuild old relationships and form new ones.

There are many benefits to making this effort. Having family and friends you can turn to gives you a sense of connection. It also provides a rich source of emotional and practical support. Your loved ones can encourage your healthy habits and remind you to stick to your treatment plan. Just knowing they are there helps reduce stress.

TALKING ABOUT YOUR ILLNESS

Opening up about your diagnosis can be difficult at first. You may be worried about how your loved ones will react to the news. In truth, while some family members and friends may be supportive right off the bat, others might not respond as well as they could. Often, bad reactions are just a matter of ignorance, and as your loved ones learn more about your illness, they'll grow more supportive.

Often, bad reactions are just a matter of ignorance, and as your loved ones learn more about your illness, they'll grow more supportive.

By now, you probably know quite a bit about schizophrenia. You and your loved ones will both benefit if you pass along your knowledge. If you're already getting treatment for your illness, be sure to mention that. If you need help to find treatment, ask for assistance as clearly and directly as you can.

It's always a good idea to keep those closest to you informed about your illness. Beyond that, it's your choice whether to tell other people, such as classmates, more distant relatives, or friends you only see occasionally. In a perfect world, telling someone you have schizophrenia would be no different than telling them you have diabetes or asthma. In reality, some people have stereotypes about schizophrenia that might cause them to see you in an unfairly negative light.

If you suspect that less-close acquaintances might not be supportive, there's no reason you have to discuss your illness with them. On the other hand, you might feel that the only way to fight stereotypes is to be open and set the record straight about their misconceptions. The decision is up to you.

MAKING AND KEEPING FRIENDS

Schizophrenia often makes it more difficult to get acquainted with other people. You might have trouble expressing your thoughts and feelings, or you might have a hard time understanding the viewpoints of others. Be patient with the process. Like anything else, making friends gets easier with practice.

One thing that's certain: You can't make friends sitting alone in your room. Get out and become involved in community activities. That's the best way to meet people who share your interests, which is the seed out of which many friendships grow. These are some ideas for meeting people:

- Strike up a conversation with students who sit next to you in class.
- Join an afterschool group or a community club related to your hobby.
- Volunteer at your school, church, synagogue, or community center.

- Sign up for a sport through your school or a local sports league.

While activities are important, don't take on more than you can do. Be sure to leave some time in your schedule for relaxing and recharging. One key to a healthy lifestyle is balancing activity with rest.

Another good way to find friends is by joining a self-help group. When you're feeling down, you can find encouragement in someone else's recovery. When you're feeling overwhelmed, you can get coping tips from other people who have dealt with similar challenges. And when you're feeling proud of your accomplishments, you can share your successes with the group.

DATING AND PHYSICAL INTIMACY

Dating can be fun and exciting, but it also may make you feel nervous and stressed at times. Such mixed feelings are normal, whether or not you have schizophrenia, but you still might want to discuss them with your treatment provider. Your provider can offer helpful suggestions on handling the strong feelings that dating can stir up.

One decision you may face is whether or not to become physically intimate with the person you're dating. This is a big step, so it needs to be considered carefully, not made on the spur of the moment. If you're in a long-term, caring relationship and thinking about taking this step, you might want to discuss it first with a parent, your health care provider, a clergyperson, or another older person whose advice you trust.

Be aware that schizophrenia itself as well as the medications used to treat it sometimes affect sexual desire and performance. In both males and females, lack of sexual desire and enjoyment are common problems. Some males also have problems getting and maintaining erections. If you're having sexual difficulties that distress you, talk to your doctor about them. While you might feel a little embarrassed or uncomfortable, keep in mind that sexuality is a normal part of life and something that your doctor is accustomed to discussing.

How Not to Become a Crime Victim

One stereotype about schizophrenia is that it's linked to crime. While there's a grain of truth in this statement, the reality is that people with schizophrenia are much more likely to be the victims than the offenders.

An eye-opening recent study compared 936 patients with severe mental illness to more than 32,000 people from the general population. Over one-quarter of the patients had been victims of an attempted or completed violent crime within the past year, a rate more than 11 times higher than the comparison group. The patients also were 4 times more likely than the comparison group to have been victims of a property crime, and 140 times more likely to have experienced personal theft. While these numbers are staggering, they may actually be underestimates, since the patients in the study were all receiving treatment. It's likely that people with severe mental illness who aren't getting care are even easier prey for criminals.

Protect yourself from becoming a crime statistic. These steps can help:

- Find a safe place to spend your free time. You're much less likely to become a crime victim at a peer support center than on the street.
- Be cautious about displaying money or other items that someone might want to steal—such as a cell phone or jewelry—when in public.
- Pay attention to your surroundings when walking down the street. Stay in well-lighted areas with other people around.
- Be aware of the distinction between taking sensible precautions and having paranoid thoughts that cause you to go overboard. To sort out the difference, talk to your treatment provider about any safety concerns.

Remember that you also have a right to say "no" if you don't feel ready for sexual activity. Don't be afraid to stand up for yourself. Unfortunately, even if you say "no" clearly and directly, it's possible you might run into someone who won't respect your wishes. To minimize this risk, avoid getting into situations that leave you vulnerable to unwanted advances or sexual assault. It's safer and often more comfortable to go out in a group and confine your dates to public places.

What Are Tips for Coping With Stress and Change?

Stress and change are inevitable, and they aren't necessarily bad. A little stress and change can spice up your life, assuming you manage them effectively. However, in people with schizophrenia, too much stress may make delusions and hallucinations worse. In addition, prolonged stress can create new problems, contributing to a host of physical and psychological ailments—everything from anxiety, depression, and irritability to heart disease, digestive disorders, and frequent infections.

Finding effective ways to manage stress is a critical part of living well with schizophrenia. Some sources of stress can be avoided. For instance, if keeping up with the demands of four classes is causing too much pressure, you could cut back to just three. If living with a noisy roommate is creating constant friction, you could look for a new roommate. If you're feeling stressed by boredom and inactivity, you could join a club and start taking daily walks.

Finding effective ways to manage stress is a critical part of living well with schizophrenia.

Other sources of stress aren't so easily eliminated. To manage them, you need to learn how to counter stress by relaxing your body and calming your mind. Different strategies are effective for different people, so experiment to find what works best for you. Here are some suggestions:

- Talk about what's bothering you. The longer you keep your feelings bottled up, the more likely it is they'll come out in inappropriate ways, such as withdrawing from other people, getting into arguments, or abusing alcohol or other drugs. Talking about problems as they arise helps keep pressure from building up to a dangerous level. It also gives you a chance to ask for assistance, which may help you solve problems sooner rather than later.
- Change how you look at change. Instead of regarding new demands as threats, try to see them as opportunities to learn skills and show what you can do. A therapist may be able to help you work on replacing self-defeating, negative thoughts with more constructive, positive ones.
- Make exercise part of your daily routine. Exercise—such as walking, swimming, or cycling—is a great stress reliever. It also enhances your sense of well-being and gives you something to look forward to. Plus, it helps control the weight gain that is a side effect of some medications.
- Learn some methods of relaxing. One simple way to relax quickly is by taking a series of slow, deep breaths while you focus on the air moving in and out. Some people also like to imagine a relaxing scene or listen to soothing music. Find what works for you and practice it on a regular basis.

Many people feel hopeless when first diagnosed with schizophrenia. They may envision a bleak future marked by the loss of their dreams. Fortunately, it doesn't have to be that way. Proper treatment and rehabilitation coupled with a healthy lifestyle can go a long way toward managing symptoms and maximizing recovery.

There is life after schizophrenia. And it can be a very good one.

Chapter Six

Putting the Pieces Back Together:
My Life Today

Epilogue to My Story

I continue to take medication as prescribed. Medication is the reason I was able to recover. I had lived with delusions for years and never recognized the fallacy of my beliefs until I started taking it.

It has now been more than six years since I first started taking antipsychotic drugs. I've had a few unpleasant side effects over the years, but these were managed effectively with the help of my doctors. Now, I experience side effects infrequently, if at all. The improvement in my mental status has been gradual but continuous, and I have not had any clinical symptoms of schizophrenia for at least four years. I also seem to be progressing in other ways that are not easily classified by a doctor. My productivity at work and my outlook on life all seem to improve as time passes. Most people who meet me now would find it hard to believe that I ever had a mental illness. Many people are surprised when I tell them I have schizophrenia.

I now talk openly about my disease. Nearly everyone I work with knows about it, and I've also told several people in the fire department. They don't seem to treat me any differently and

I have found that sharing my past problems with friends and co-workers has made us closer.

they accept me for who I am. I have found that sharing my past problems with friends and co-workers has made us closer. I haven't been alienated as you might think. Of course, I am not expressing any symptoms of the disease and I am sure the absence of these symptoms affects their opinion of me.

The improvement in my life is not entirely due to medication, though. I was lucky to have the continuous support of my friends and family. My roommates (with whom I shared a house until I became psychotic) forgave my overdue rent. My parents allowed me to live at their house while I was ill (actually, they demanded that I live there). Dan and Helen have continued to offer me steady emotional support, even though I rejected them during my illness, and Dan helped me to kickstart a new career by providing me with financial support. Another friend gave me numerous reference books to help with my education, and he supported me by hiring me to do some handyman chores that he could have done himself.

I was also recommended for my current job by someone who knew I had schizophrenia. This person didn't stereotype me as a lifelong lunatic. After I got the job, my boss allowed me some time off work when I was experiencing heavy anxiety. My fellow members of the fire department who know about my illness have pushed me forward and encouraged me to assume more responsibility as the years have passed. I'm now their president!

Don't be ashamed to accept help from anyone. No one can be successful in recovering from a serious illness like schizophrenia without the help and support of others.

Try not to be impatient when measuring your improvement. All of my progress has been gradual. Success doesn't come fast. Anyone with serious mental illness must realize this. Give yourself a chance. You may be having serious problems now, but things can slowly improve. Don't try to achieve too much too soon because you may overextend yourself. Set small goals, and try to make small improvements in your life. Over time, they add up to big improvements.

> Set small goals, and try to make small improvements in your life.

Also realize that there are setbacks to treatment. I experienced several discouraging problems—depression, anxiety, and weight gain to name a few. Working closely with your doctor, you may be able to work through these setbacks, or keep them to a minimum. Don't give up. Most importantly, take the medication and report *any* problems to your doctor. Schizophrenia is an illness that must be taken seriously and needs to be managed for life. If you have schizophrenia, don't stop treatment when you are feeling better because it's the treatment that makes you feel better! Also, don't stop treatment if you are feeling worse—you need to work out these problems with your doctor's assistance.

If you cannot afford treatment, ask your doctor, your pharmacist, and your government health department about special plans that help you pay for treatment. Don't be too proud to accept financial assistance from any source, be it government programs, scholarships, or the help of family and friends. You can always find some way to repay this generosity when you are stronger. In my case, I relied upon a government-subsidized prescription plan to pay for my medication for more than a year. Find a way to continue your treatment no matter what!

Keep up the hope. Look to the future, not to the past. Good luck!

Frequently Asked Questions

Making Treatment Decisions

I know I need help, but I'm not sure where to start looking for it. Any suggestions?

Your parents or other older relatives are often your first, best source of assistance with finding professional help. However, other good sources include your family doctor, school counselor, school nurse, or clergyperson. If you're in college, the student counseling center probably won't offer the type of treatment you need for schizophrenia, but may be able to direct you to other treatment resources on campus or in the community. The employee assistance program at your or your parent's job can do the same. In addition, the federal government's Center for Mental Health Services offers a free, online directory of mental health service providers around the country (mentalhealth.samhsa.gov/databases).

I'm already in treatment, but I'm not satisfied with the care I'm getting. What can I do?

First, make sure that your expectations are realistic. As time goes on, you should feel comfortable with your treatment provider and be able to trust that he or she is acting in your best interest. Your distress should gradually diminish, while your self-assurance and ability to get along in everyday life should slowly grow. That being said, treatment for schizophrenia takes months or years, not days, and it requires a real effort on your part. If you're giving it your best shot, and you still feel that you aren't getting adequate results, talk to your provider about your concerns. A good provider will welcome this type of feedback and respond to your feelings. If you've tried this step and are still dissatisfied, you might want to set up a consultation with another provider who can help you decide whether it's time to seek a new doctor or therapist.

Living With Schizophrenia

How can I control my weight now that I'm taking medication for schizophrenia?

Weight gain is a common side effect of antipsychotic medications. Clozapine and olanzapine are notorious for producing large gains of 15 pounds or more, but other medications can lead to weight gain, too. A sensible diet and regular exercise are critical for managing this problem and promoting good health. Experts recommend a diet composed mainly of fruits, vegetables, whole grains, and fat-free or low-fat milk and dairy products. There's also room for some lean meats, poultry, fish, beans, eggs, and nuts. While an occasional treat is okay, limit foods that are high in fat and added sugars. As far as exercise

goes, aim for at least 30 minutes of moderate-intensity physical activity on all or most days of the week. If you're trying to
lose weight rather than just keep from gaining, you may need
to exercise a little longer.

Can I treat my symptoms by taking a supplement or eating a special diet?

The healthful diet described above can help you feel better in a
general sense. However, no supplement or special diet has been
proven to be a specific treatment for symptoms of schizophrenia. Some preliminary studies suggested that eliminating
wheat and milk might help reduce the severity of symptoms in
a small percentage of schizophrenia patients, but larger studies
are needed to confirm those results. Since whole wheat foods
and low-fat or fat-free milk and dairy products are so nutri-
tious, it's important not to cut them from your diet without
talking to your doctor first. Also, keep in mind that no supplement or diet can take the place of medication and therapy.

Can I drive a car if I have schizophrenia?

There isn't a one-size-fits-all answer to this question. Some
people with schizophrenia have trouble with planning and
judgment, which might affect their ability to plan out a driving
route and make good decisions in traffic. Other people have a
problem paying attention, which obviously could be dangerous when they're behind the wheel. In addition, studies show
that antipsychotic medications can slow people's reaction time,
which could affect their ability to brake quickly or swerve
around a sudden obstacle. To sum up, driving a car takes planning, judgment, concentration, and coordination, and these
abilities can all be affected by schizophrenia or its treatment.

Before you get behind the wheel, talk to your health care provider about whether it's safe for you.

Schizophrenia In Society

Is it true that people with schizophrenia are often violent?

The public perception that people with schizophrenia pose a danger to others has been fed by intense media coverage of a few isolated yet tragically memorable events, such as the death of a young woman who was pushed in front of a New York City subway by a man with untreated schizophrenia. As a group, though, people with schizophrenia who are receiving proper treatment are no more likely to behave violently than people without the disease. A small subset of those with schizophrenia seem to be at risk for becoming violent. However, this risk can be minimized if they take their medication as prescribed and avoid abusing alcohol or other drugs. In truth, the vast majority of violent crimes are committed by people who *don't* have a mental illness.

What's the relationship between schizophrenia and homelessness?

An estimated 20% to 25% of homeless individuals have a serious mental illness such as schizophrenia. They often have active, untreated symptoms, which makes it very difficult for them to seek out the help they need. Many also abuse alcohol or other drugs, and most have lost touch with family members. Without public assistance, homeless individuals with schizophrenia sometimes end up living on the streets for years. Yet when given the opportunity, most can benefit from treatment, housing, and support services. To learn more about this important issue, visit the websites of the National Resource and Training Center on Homelessness and Mental Illness (www.nrchmi.samhsa.gov) and the National Coalition for the Homeless (www.nationalhomeless.org).

Fighting Stigma and Stereotypes

What does being mentally ill really mean?

A mental illness is nothing more than a brain disorder that affects your thoughts, moods, emotions, or complex behaviors, such as interacting with other people or planning future activities. In reality, having a mental illness is no different from having a disorder that affects your heart, lungs, muscles, or bones. Unfortunately, not everyone understands this simple fact. Some people mistakenly associate having a mental illness with being weak or dangerous. Because mental illness is such an emotionally charged term, you might sometimes feel more comfortable referring to schizophrenia as a brain disorder instead. That's totally up to you, however. Both terms are equally accurate.

How should I react when other people make hurtful comments?

Remind yourself that their behavior reflects on them, not on you. At the very least, it tells you that they are uninformed. It's a common problem. According to a 2006 survey sponsored by the U.S. Department of Health and Human Services, only about one-fourth of young adults ages 18 to 24 believe that a person with mental illness can recover, and fewer than half of Americans believe that someone with mental illness can be as successful as anyone else at work. The best antidote to such stereotypes is the truth. Look the person in the eye and briefly state your case in a calm voice. A firm yet polite response is usually all it takes to set the record straight. But if the other person continues to make belittling or mean-spirited remarks, simply walk away. There's no reason you should have to put up with verbal abuse or disrespect.

What else can I do to spread the word about schizophrenia?

If you're interested in fighting stigma and promoting change on a broader scale, consider volunteering for an organization such as the National Alliance on Mental Illness (NAMI, 800-950-6264, www.nami.org) or National Mental Health Association (800-969-6642, www.nmha.org). Both of these organizations have active advocacy programs that strive to influence public policy at a local, state, and national level. There are a variety of ways to get involved, including writing lawmakers, talking to the media, giving presentations, and participating in fundraisers. By making your voice heard, you put society on notice that people with schizophrenia are a positive force to be reckoned with.

Glossary

affect   A person's changing emotional state.

agranulocytosis   A disorder in which bone marrow doesn't produce enough white blood cells to fight infection. It is a potential side effect of Clozaril (clozapine).

alogia   A reduction in the quantity or quality of speech.

Americans with Disabilities Act (ADA)   A federal law that gives civil rights protections to individuals with disabilities. Protections are similar to those provided to individuals on the basis of race, color, sex, national origin, age, and religion.

anhedonia   A loss of interest or pleasure in activities that a person once enjoyed.

antipsychotic   A drug used to treat the symptoms of schizophrenia.

assertive community treatment (ACT)   A treatment approach for people with the most severe and long-lasting mental illness. A team of professionals works together to provide comprehensive treatment and supports that are tailored to the individual's needs.

atypical antipsychotic   One of the newer antipsychotic medications.

auditory hallucination   Hearing something that no one else can hear. This type of hallucination usually takes the form of hearing voices.

avolition   A pervasive lack of initiative and motivation.

behavior therapy   A form of therapy that focuses on changing or replacing unwanted behaviors.

case management   A service designed to access and coordinate all the different treatments and services a particular individual receives.

catatonic schizophrenia   A type of schizophrenia characterized by severe disturbances in movement and a marked lack of responsiveness to the outside world.

clubhouse   A place where people with mental illness can slowly adjust to a work-centered day, first by doing the jobs needed to run the clubhouse and then by taking short-term jobs in the community.

cognitive symptoms   Deficits in thinking ability as a result of schizophrenia, such as problems with making decisions, paying attention, and remembering.

cognitive therapy   A form of therapy that focuses on correcting inaccurate patterns of thinking.

deinstitutionalization   A movement that led to the widespread release of individuals from mental institutions.

delusion   A false personal belief that has no basis in reality and remains unchanged even when the person is presented with strong evidence to the contrary.

delusion of grandeur   An irrational and highly exaggerated sense of one's own power, knowledge, or special relationship to God or a famous person.

delusion of persecution   An irrational belief that one is being plotted against, spied upon, followed, tricked, or harassed.

depot medication   A special type of injection that releases the medication slowly over a period of weeks.

disorganized schizophrenia   A type of schizophrenia characterized by disorganized speech and behavior along with flat or inappropriate affect.

dissociative identity disorder   A mental disorder in which a person has two or more distinct identities that take turns controlling his or her behavior. Also called multiple personality disorder.

dopamine   A neurotransmitter that is essential for movement and also influences motivation and perception of reality.

electroencephalogram (EEG)   A diagnostic technique that produces a graphic record of electrical activity within the brain.

family psychoeducation   A program that helps family members partner with the person who has a mental illness so they all can work together toward recovery.

family therapy   A form of talk therapy in which several members of a family participate in therapy sessions together.

flat affect   An extreme lack of any signs of emotional expression.

gamma-amino-butyric acid (GABA)   A neurotransmitter that inhibits the flow of nerve signals in neurons by blocking the release of other neurotransmitters.

glutamate   A neurotransmitter that promotes the flow of nerve signals in neurons.

group therapy   A form of talk therapy in which a group of people with similar problems work on specific issues together under the guidance of a therapist.

hallucination   A false sensory impression, in which the person sees, hears, smells, tastes, or feels something that isn't really there.

hippocampus   A brain structure involved in emotion, learning, and memory.

illness management training   A program geared to helping people with mental illness develop personal strategies for coping with their disease.

individualized education program (IEP)   A written educational plan for a student who qualifies for services under the Individuals with Disabilities Education Improvement Act of 2004.

Individuals with Disabilities Education Improvement Act (IDEA)   A federal law that applies to students who have a disability that impacts their ability to benefit from general educational services.

magnetic resonance imaging (MRI)   A powerful imaging technique that uses magnets and radio waves to produce pictures of body organs and tissues.

major depression   A disorder that involves being in a low mood nearly all the time, or losing interest or enjoyment in almost everything. These feelings last for at least two weeks and cause significant distress or problems in everyday life.

managed care   A system designed to keep the cost of health care down.

Medicaid   A joint federal-state government program that provides health insurance to eligible low-income and disabled individuals.

mood stabilizer   A medication that helps even out severe mood swings.

negative symptoms   Normal emotions and behaviors that are reduced by schizophrenia and often involve a gradual withdrawal from the world.

neuroleptic malignant syndrome   A nervous system problem that can affect the kidneys. It is an uncommon but serious side effect of antipsychotic medications.

neuron   A nerve cell that is specially designed to send information to other nerve, muscle, or gland cells.

neurotransmitter   A chemical that acts as a messenger within the brain.

obsessive-compulsive disorder (OCD)   A mental disorder characterized by repeated, uncontrollable thoughts that cause anxiety as well as repetitive actions that the person feels driven to perform in response to these thoughts.

occupational therapy   The health care field that helps patients with long-term diseases learn the skills they need for daily living.

panic attack   A sudden, unexpected wave of intense fear and apprehension that is accompanied by physical symptoms, such as a racing or pounding heart, shortness of breath, and sweating. OCD is characterized by repeated, uncontrollable thoughts that cause anxiety as well as repetitive actions that the person feels driven to perform in response to the thoughts.

paranoid schizophrenia   A type of schizophrenia characterized by prominent delusions and/or frequent auditory hallucinations. The delusions often involve being persecuted by others.

partial hospitalization   A treatment option where the person spends at least four hours a day on therapy and other treatment-related services, but goes home at night. A wide range of services may be provided, such as individual or group therapy, special education, job training, and therapeutic recreation.

peer support center   A safe place where people with mental illness can drop in to socialize as well as find informal support and help.

positive symptoms   Abnormal perceptions, thoughts, and behaviors that are produced by schizophrenia and usually represent a break with reality.

prefrontal cortex   Part of the brain involved in complex thought, problem solving, and emotion.

prodromal symptoms   Preliminary symptoms of schizophrenia that may occur two to six years before the first major episode.

psychiatrist   A medical doctor who specializes in the diagnosis and treatment of mental illnesses and emotional problems.

psychologist   A mental health professional who provides assessment and treatment for mental and emotional disorders.

psychosis   Positive symptoms of schizophrenia, especially delusions and hallucinations.

psychosocial rehabilitation   Programs that provide psychological, social, and job training, which help individuals with mental illness regain any life skills lost due to their illness as well as develop new skills for managing their disease. Also called psychiatric rehabilitation.

psychotic break   Loss of contact with reality as a result of schizophrenia.

reasonable accommodation   An adjustment to a job or the work environment that enables a qualified person with a disability to perform the essential functions of his or her job.

receptor   A molecule that recognizes a specific chemical, such as a neurotransmitter. For a chemical message to be sent from one nerve cell to another, the message must be delivered to a matching receptor on the surface of the receiving nerve cell.

recreational therapy   The health care field that uses activities such as arts and crafts, games, dance, movement, and music to improve overall well-being and help patients hone their social skills.

relapse   A return of symptoms after a period of improvement.

residential treatment center   A treatment facility where the person lives in a dorm-like setting with a small group of people. The treatment there is less specialized and intensive than in a hospital, but the stay may last considerably longer.

schizoaffective disorder   A mental disorder that combines the distorted thoughts and perceptions of schizophrenia with severe disturbances in mood.

schizophrenia   A severe, long-lasting mental disorder that produces symptoms such as distorted thoughts and perceptions, disorganized speech and behavior, and a reduced ability to feel emotions.

Section 504   A section of the Rehabilitation Act that applies to students who have a physical or mental impairment that substantially limits one or more major life activity.

self-help group   A group that brings together people with a common concern so they can share support, encouragement, and hands-on advice.

serotonin   A neurotransmitter that helps regulate mood, sleep, appetite, and sexual drive.

social skills training   A program that helps people with schizophrenia develop the skills they need to communicate effectively and interact well with others.

State Child Health Insurance Program (SCHIP)   A joint federal-state government program that provides health insurance for the children in certain lower-income families who aren't eligible for Medicaid.

supported employment   A service that helps people with mental illness find and keep jobs in the community that pay at least minimum wage and are suited to their interests and abilities.

supportive therapy   A form of talk therapy in which the goal is to strengthen people's coping skills and provide them with reassurance.

synapse   The gap between two nerve cells that serves as the site where information is relayed from one cell to the next.

tardive dyskinesia   A disorder causing repeated, involuntary, purposeless movements that sometimes develops after long-term use of antipsychotic medications, especially the older ones.

typical antipsychotic   One of the older antipsychotic medications.

utilization review   A formal review of health care services to determine whether payment for them should be authorized or denied.

ventricles   Fluid-filled cavities inside the brain.

Resources

Organizations

American Academy of Child and Adolescent Psychiatry
3615 Wisconsin Ave. NW
Washington, DC 20016
(202) 966-7300
www.aacap.org
www.parentsmedguide.org

American Psychiatric Association
1000 Wilson Blvd., Suite 1825
Arlington, VA 22209
(888) 357-7924
www.psych.org
www.healthyminds.org
www.parentsmedguide.org

American Psychological Association
750 First St. NE
Washington, DC 20002
(800) 374-2721
www.apa.org
www.apahelpcenter.org
www.psychologymatters.org

Assertive Community Treatment Association
810 E. Grand River Ave., Suite 102
Brighton, MI 48116

(810) 227-1859
www.actassociation.org

International Center for Clubhouse Development
425 West 47th St.
New York, NY 10036
(212) 582-0343
www.iccd.org

NARSAD, The National Mental Health Research Association
60 Cutter Mill Rd., Suite 404
Great Neck, NY 11021
(800) 829-8289
www.narsad.org

National Alliance on Mental Illness
Colonial Place Three
2107 Wilson Blvd., Suite 300
Arlington, VA 22201
(800) 950-6264
www.nami.org

National Institute of Mental Health
6001 Executive Blvd., Room 8184, MSC 9663
Bethesda, MD 20892
(866) 615-6464
www.nimh.nih.gov

National Mental Health Association
2001 N. Beauregard St., 12th Floor
Alexandria, VA 22311
(800) 969-6642
www.nmha.org

National Mental Health Consumers' Self-Help Clearinghouse
1211 Chestnut St., Suite 1207
Philadelphia, PA 19107
(800) 553-4539
www.mhselfhelp.org
www.cdsdirectory.org

National Mental Health Information Center
P.O. Box 42557
Washington, DC 20015

(800) 789-2647
www.mentalhealth.samhsa.gov

National Schizophrenia Foundation
403 Seymour Ave., Suite 202
Lansing, Michigan 48933
(800) 482-9534
www.nsfoundation.org

World Fellowship for Schizophrenia and Allied Disorders
124 Merton St., Suite 507
Toronto, Ontario, M4S 2Z2
Canada
(416) 961-2855
www.world-schizophrenia.org

Educational Issues

Individuals with Disabilities Education Improvement Act of 2004
U.S. Department of Education
Office of Special Education and Rehabilitative Services
400 Maryland Ave. SW
Washington, DC 20202
(800) 872-5327
www.ed.gov/idea

Office for Civil Rights
U.S. Department of Education
550 12th St. SW
Washington, DC 20202-1100
(800) 421-3481
www.ed.gov/ocr

Parent Advocacy Coalition for Educational Rights
8161 Normandale Blvd.
Minneapolis, MN 55437
(952) 838-9000
www.pacer.org

Employment Issues

Americans with Disabilities Act
U.S. Department of Justice

Civil Rights Division, Disability Rights Section
950 Pennsylvania Ave. NW
Washington, DC 20530
(800) 514-0301
www.ada.gov

Job Accommodation Network
U.S. Department of Labor
Office of Disability Employment Policy
P.O. Box 6080
Morgantown, WV 26506
(800) 526-7234
www.jan.wvu.edu

Legal Issues (General)

Bazelon Center for Mental Health Law
1101 15th St. NW, Suite 1212
Washington, DC 20005
(202) 467-5730
www.bazelon.org

National Disability Rights Network
900 Second St. NE, Suite 211
Washington, DC 20002
(202) 408-9514
www.napas.org

Books

DeLisi, Lynn E. *100 Questions & Answers About Schizophrenia: Painful Minds.* Sudbury, MA: Johns and Bartlett, 2006.
Frith, Christopher, and Eve Johnstone. *Schizophrenia: A Very Short Introduction.* New York: Oxford University Press, 2003.
Miller, Rachel, and Susan E. Mason. *Diagnosis Schizophrenia: A Comprehensive Resource.* New York: Columbia University Press, 2002.
Torrey, E. Fuller. *Surviving Schizophrenia: A Manual for Families, Consumers, and Providers* (4th ed.). New York: HarperCollins, 2001.

First-Person Accounts

McLean, Richard. *Recovered, Not Cured.* Crows Nest, Australia: Allen & Unwin, 2003.

Steele, Ken, and Claire Berman. *The Day the Voices Stopped: A Memoir of Madness and Hope.* New York: Basic Books, 2001.

Wagner, Pamela Spiro, and Carolyn S. Spiro. *Divided Minds: Twin Sisters and Their Journey Through Schizophrenia.* New York: St. Martin's Press, 2005.

Biographical Accounts

Nasar, Sylvia. *A Beautiful Mind.* New York: Simon & Schuster, 1998.

Web Sites

Evidence-Based Practices Shaping Mental Health Services Toward Recovery, Center for Mental Health Services and the Robert Wood Johnson Foundation, www.mentalhealthpractices.org

HUBIN: Human Brain Informatics, Karolinska Institute Department of Clinical Neuroscience, www.hubin.org/index_en.html

MindZone, Annenberg Foundation Trust at Sunnylands with the Annenberg Public Policy Center of the University of Pennsylvania, www.CopeCareDeal.org

New York City Voices, www.newyorkcityvoices.org

Help for Related Problems

Anxiety Disorders

ORGANIZATIONS

Anxiety Disorders Association of America, (240) 485-1001, www.adaa.org

Freedom From Fear, (718) 351-1717, www.freedomfromfear.org

Obsessive-Compulsive Foundation, (203) 401-2070, www.ocfoundation.org

BOOKS

Ford, Emily, with Michael R. Liebowitz, M.D., and Linda Wasmer Andrews. *What You Must Think of Me: A Firsthand Account of One Teenager's Experience With Social Anxiety Disorder.* New York: Oxford University Press with the Annenberg Foundation Trust at Sunnylands and the Annenberg Public Policy Center at the University of Pennsylvania, 2007.

Kant, Jared, with Martin Franklin, Ph.D., and Linda Wasmer Andrews. *The Thought That Counts: A Firsthand Account of One Teenager's Experience With Obsessive-Compulsive Disorder.* New York: Oxford University Press with the Annenberg Foundation Trust at Sunnylands and the Annenberg Public Policy Center at the University of Pennsylvania, forthcoming in 2008.

Mood Disorders

ORGANIZATIONS

Child and Adolescent Bipolar Foundation, (847) 256-8525, www.cabf.org

Depression and Bipolar Support Alliance, (800) 826-3632, www.dbsalliance.org

Depression and Related Affective Disorders Association, (410) 583-2919, www
.drada.org

Families for Depression Awareness, (781) 890-0220, www.familyaware.org

BOOKS

Irwin, Cait, with Dwight L. Evans, M.D., and Linda Wasmer Andrews. *Mono-chrome Days: A Firsthand Account of One Teenager's Experience With Depression.* New York: Oxford University Press with the Annenberg Foundation Trust at Sunnylands and the Annenberg Public Policy Center at the University of Pennsylvania, 2007.

Jamieson, Patrick E., Ph.D., with Moira A. Rynn Ph.D. *Mind Race: A Firsthand Account of One Teenager's Experience With Bipolar Disorder.* New York: Oxford University Press with the Annenberg Foundation Trust at Sunnylands and the Annenberg Public Policy Center at the University of Pennsylvania, 2006.

Substance Abuse

ORGANIZATIONS

Alcoholics Anonymous, (212) 870-3400 (check your phone book for a local number), www.aa.org

American Council for Drug Education, (800) 488-3784, www.acde.org

Narcotics Anonymous, (818) 773-9999, www.na.org

National Council on Alcoholism and Drug Dependence, (800) 622-2255, www.ncadd.org

National Institute on Alcohol Abuse and Alcoholism, (301) 443–3860, www
.niaaa.nih.gov, www.collegedrinkingprevention.gov

National Institute on Drug Abuse, (301) 443-1124, www.drugabuse.gov, teens
.drugabuse.gov

Partnership for a Drug-Free America, (212) 922-1560, www.drugfreeamerica.com

Substance Abuse and Mental Health Services Administration, (800) 729-6686, ncadi.samhsa.gov, csat.samhsa.gov, prevention.samhsa.gov

BOOK

Keegan, Kyle, with Howard B. Moss, M.D., *Chasing the High: A Firsthand Account of One Young Person's Experience With Substance Abuse.* New York: Oxford University Press with the Annenberg Foundation Trust at Sunnylands and the

Annenberg Public Policy Center at the University of Pennsylvania, forthcoming in 2008.

WEB SITES

Facts on Tap, Phoenix House, www.factsontap.org

Freevibe, National Youth Anti-Drug Media Campaign, www.freevibe.com

The New Science of Addiction: Genetics and the Brain, Genetic Science Learning Center at the University of Utah, gslc.genetics.utah.edu/units/addiction

Suicidal Thoughts

ORGANIZATIONS

American Foundation for Suicide Prevention, (888) 333-2377, www.afsp.org

Jed Foundation, (212) 647-7544, www.jedfoundation.org

Suicide Awareness Voices of Education, (952) 946-7998, www.save.org

Suicide Prevention Action Network USA, (202) 449-3600, www.spanusa.org

BOOK

Lezine, DeQuincy A., Ph.D., and David Brent, M.D. *Eight Stories Up: An Adolescent Chooses Hope Over Suicide.* New York: Oxford University Press with the Annenberg Foundation Trust at Sunnylands and the Annenberg Public Policy Center at the University of Pennsylvania, forthcoming in 2008.

HOTLINES

National Hopeline Network, (800) 784-2433, www.hopeline.com

National Suicide Prevention Lifeline, (800) 273-8255, www.suicideprevention lifeline.org

Bibliography

American Psychiatric Association. *Diagnostic and Statistical Manual of Mental Disorders* (4th ed., text revision). Washington, DC: American Psychiatric Association, 2000.

Bellack, Alan S., Kim T. Mueser, Susan Gingerich, and Julie Agresta. *Social Skills Training for Schizophrenia: A Step-by-Step Guide* (2nd ed.). New York: Guilford Press, 2004.

Evans, Dwight L., Edna B. Foa, Raquel E. Gur, Herbert Hendin, Charles P. O'Brien, Martin E. P. Seligman, and B. Timothy Walsh (Eds.). *Treating and Preventing Adolescent Mental Health Disorders: What We Know and What We Don't Know.* New York: Oxford University Press with the Annenberg Foundation Trust at Sunnylands and the Annenberg Public Policy Center of the University of Pennsylvania, 2005.

Green, Michael Foster. *Schizophrenia Revealed: From Neurons to Social Interactions.* New York: W.W. Norton: 2003.

Gur, Raquel E., and Ann Braden Johnson. *If Your Adolescent Has Schizophrenia: An Essential Resource for Parents.* New York: Oxford University Press with the Annenberg Foundation Trust at Sunnylands and the Annenberg Public Policy Center at the University of Pennsylvania, 2006.

Index

Note: Page numbers followed by "*t*" refer to text boxes or tables.